MW01047717

CA CA

(THE IRREPRESSIBLE) AUTHENTIC M

Authentic M Productions, LLC

Copyright © 2019 by (The Irrepressible) Authentic M

All rights reserved.

No part of this book may be reproduced in any form or by any electronic or mechanical means, including information storage and retrieval systems, without written permission from the author, except for the use of brief quotations in a book review.

ISBN: 978-1-7336508-0-9

THE POOP SCOOP (CONTENTS)

"I'm a human mullet!" I once said among friends and family while dressed in a classy black blouse on top (business) with distressed jeans rolled up and black Vans on my feet (party/casual). There were a few chuckles, but really, what you see is what you get. I've come to accept the duality or perhaps complex contradictions that can exist in oneself, just as a single event may elicit a response of thank you, I'm sorry, and you're welcome.

PREFACE

Creatively Constipated

As this begins, I have no idea what is on the cover, the jacket synopsis, or what wild rave reviews have been written about the content. I suspect you may be intrigued by the concept of someone writing about poop of some variety. Let's face it, poop is funny. Everyone does it.

There are countless names for poop, pooping, or poopy situations. Think of the synonyms for poop: BM, bowel movement, ca-ca, crap, defecate, deuce, doo-doo, doody, droppings, dung, excrement, fecal matter, feces, make a stinky, manure, number two, stool, turd, and waste. I'm sure the list could go on and on, but I'll stop there. The one poop word not mentioned is the big doody of the turd world, a big no-no for most social situations: the s-word, shit.

If you think about it, most poop phrases usually use the s-word. My apologies in advance, I use curse words in real life, often out of frustration, pain, or anger. If foul language upsets your delicate sensibilities, give this book to someone else to summarize for you or edit. It won't be as funny, but that's on you. And let's face it—you've already read the word *shit* and from here on out, it's really just a repeat.

Now that we've got all that shit out of the way, we'll get down to business (Ha! Another poop phrase!). Why is this book in your hands right now? Maybe you're related to me or a friend who wanted to be supportive; thank you. Maybe you really wanted a book about poop (if so, you may be disappointed, as this chapter has the most poop references in the entire book). On the other hand, perhaps you were directed to give this book a read because it matters to you or someone you know, and it contains something you need or can relate to in your life. Regardless of how you came to hold this book, I welcome you to my story.

So why should you read a book titled *CA CA*? Usually ca-ca is another word for poop. But take another look at the title and you will not find a *little* ca-ca, but a *BIG CA CA*. What is *CA CA*? A big poop? Not in this case. "CA" is an abbreviation. California, maybe? Nope, never been there, though I do hope to go one day (Hi Ellen!). The "CA" I'm referring to is nothing like a vacation by the beach—it is the medical abbreviation for cancer. I think we can all agree that cancer is without question *shitty*.

So why *CA CA*? The simplest explanation is that I've had cancer twice, and also the thought of a title with a double meaning just struck me as funny. My close friends and family know I have a corny sense of humor. I can be silly at times, able to whip out parody songs in minutes, as well as some inappropriate or dark humor. It's a coping mechanism really. I love to hear people laugh and to put them at ease. That shtick of mine comes in handy on the job, making tough days easier for coworkers and patients. What you are reading now has taken years to develop and refine thanks to my family, friends, and life situations.

I'm a relatively young cancer survivor who also happens to be a registered nurse. There is so much information given about diagnosis, treatment, appointments, medications, side effects, as well as financial and work obligations. There might be times when people (such as medical personnel, support staff, employers, insurance carriers, and various others) assume you know details or forget to tell you about them. Some of those are small in the great scheme of things, while others are rather significant and assist in making life-altering decisions. I've interacted with enough people to know there are misconceptions about cancer and cancer patients by family, friends, coworkers, and even people in the medical field. It's time to get really honest about two words that make people uncomfortable when used separately or in combination: breast cancer.

Why do I feel compelled to share my experiences and private thoughts? It is my hope that by exploring my situation, other patients will get a heads up about cancer treatment and also validation that their feelings are normal. I want to enlighten caregivers to the darkness that keeps a patient awake all hours. It's a reminder to my fellow healthcare workers that patients—including me—are more than an account number or diagnosis. Let's also consider why people are so embarrassed by the word *breast* and why they allow crass marketing of deadly diseases in our day and age.

In June 2011, I'd written a little bit, but had slacked off since the kids finished the school year. Then a friend mailed a book across the country, a book she'd found at a library sale about someone's experience with breast cancer. I read it in one day. Although the author's experience was quite different from mine, reading it was a sign for me to tell it like it is in my own writing. By text, I sent my friend a thank you and told her how meaningful the gift was to my own writing. Her response was "Right on momma, be your authentic self!" That's how Authentic M came about as my pen name (or what I'll use if I ever become a rapper, in case you wondered).

If this little creation of mine goes further than my own

computer or the email accounts of my closest confidants, it has to be the real me, authentic in every way and told in my voice. And at this point in life, I tend to write like I speak and I promise to tell it like it is.

So turn the page and let's get this shit started.

SHIT HAPPENS

"What's this?" my husband asked, in the midst of spooning, his hand having grazed my right breast and abruptly stopped.

I followed his hand to the area, my first thought, "That's just my rib."

I sat up and felt it again. It definitely wasn't my rib. It was more like a jellybean along the lower inner edge of my right breast.

At 32 years old, no one expects to find a breast lump, especially when they have no family history of breast cancer. You can go to any number of websites, magazines, or medical texts—they'll tell you what your odds are for disease based on age, lifestyle, and family history. According to breast-cancer.org, an American woman has a 1 in 8 chance of developing breast cancer in her lifetime. They also cited a statistic that only 5-10% of breast cancers can be linked to inherited gene mutations like BRCA1 and BRCA2, but 70-80% of female breast cancer patients have no family history of breast cancer.

Think of all the people you know who have abused their

bodies (physically and chemically) and yet never seem to have consequences for their choices. Those people are the perfect example that the presence of risk factors does not guarantee a diagnosis. Likewise, a person may not have a family history of disease, but simply because they have breasts, they can develop breast cancer. That risk factor includes every man you know. Male breast cancer is rare but very real.

At my appointment with my primary care physician (PCP), we reviewed my health history and risk factors for breast cancer. They include non-smoker, average weight, active lifestyle, healthy.

Over the years, since my experience with breast cancer in 2003, I've learned of several factors that were not in my favor. One possible exposure was diethylstilbestrol (DES) in utero, which was a medication given to women to prevent miscarriage, that was later found to have the potential of producing cancer; medical professionals stopped using it in 1971 (see National Cancer Institute reference listing at the end of the book). Also, I was diagnosed with an unusual auto-immune disorder possibly related to a tick bite at 20 years old. And I was exposed to high energy radio fields while employed in radio, as well as secondhand smoke my entire life, and was on the pill (birth control) for 14 years. In addition, I also had breasts—talk about a risk factor.

It is amazing how quickly a tiny lump takes over all of your thoughts—I was seriously worried about that lump. The big squish (otherwise known as a mammogram) was scheduled within five days. The mammogram wasn't horrible, and it was definitely necessary. The results showed a mass, but an ultrasound was advised.

One week later, I returned to the outpatient diagnostic center for the breast ultrasound. The technician led me back to a dimly lit exam room. After changing out of my top and bra into a gown, I was invited to relax on a gurney where she applied warm gel onto my right breast from a squeeze bottle, and guided the probe over my breast to scan the tissue below. I didn't understand what I was seeing on the monitor but I remember the focus on a black oval that appeared on the mostly light grey image. She clicked buttons, added a location description and measurement of the mass.

My PCP's office called two days after the ultrasound, the day after Thanksgiving (side note: when have you ever been called about a medical issue the day after Thanksgiving?!?!). Happy Turkey Day... I was now scheduled for a fine needle aspiration biopsy with a local surgeon.

Everyone I talked with had an opinion, and they were all quite certain the lump was nothing.

"Can't be cancer—no family history."
"I'm sure it's not cancer; you're too young."

I met the surgeon and his staff twelve days after the ultrasound was completed. We discussed the fine needle aspiration and decided to have it done in the office. If fluid was pulled out of the lump, it was probably a cyst, which would be the easiest answer to the lump dilemma, a happy ending to all of my fears. My husband was there and we all agreed to have the procedure done in the office that day.

During the procedure, it didn't take long for the surgeon to burst my *happy ending* bubble. As I lay there on the exam table, he stated, "That is not a cyst. That—is not a cyst." He couldn't draw any fluid from the mass into the syringe.

The doctor assisted me as I sat up on the exam table, and then we discussed my options. Clearly, the lump had to come out for an up-close-and-personal meeting with a pathologist to determine what exactly it was. I was given the choice to have the procedure done that day in the office or the procedure could be scheduled at the hospital. The doctor gave my husband and me a few minutes to consider the options.

Feeling a sense of urgency, I gave the lump a speedy eviction notice and settled in for the lump removal.

We moved from the exam room to a special procedure room across the hall. I sat on the side edge of the table as instruments were gathered from cabinets and drawers by the nurse. Next I eased to my back and kept my head toward the left looking at the cabinets, trying to keep my gaze and breath away from what was going to be a surgical site. My right breast was swabbed with antiseptic, and surgical drapes were spread across my chest. The surgeon used a local anesthetic to numb the tissue and then removed the lump, sutured the incision, and applied a dressing. Based on what the surgeon found, there was a possibility that the mass was a fibroadenoma, a benign nodule, but I would have to wait for the pathology report. With all the experts still rather positive that it wasn't cancer, I settled in to wait the three days for my follow-up appointment.

My husband and I maintained our usual routine of caring for the kids, getting everyone to school or activities, and working. Our daughter (whom I shall refer to as Tink) was in third grade and very into gymnastics. Our son (we live in the South-ish—henceforth, I'll call him Bubba) was in pre-school, majoring in Hot Wheels and monster trucks, with a minor in Nintendo Gameboy. I was a full-time mom going to vocational school to be a licensed practical nurse (LPN), while working weekends as a certified medication and nurse aide. My husband worked in the city all week, then took care of the kids and household on the weekends. It was just the four of us. Before Bubba came along, we'd moved to the middle of the country from the East Coast after my husband got out of the Air Force. We had no family nearby to drop the kids with for date night or sick days from school. That time in our lives sounds crazy busy and it was—one might say stressful. Now let's add a pesky breast lump to the mix.

Couldn't be cancer.

Shouldn't be cancer.

Five days, a week, twelve days, and three more days—nearly a month—and I was about to know what was going on with my breast. Sometimes I'm a "details" person and can recall events very clearly. It was a rather nice December afternoon for Oklahoma. I remember arriving to the appointment and being put into a room to wait for the surgeon. There were other rooms with patients ahead of me. Doors opened and closed. I heard muted conversations, and then everything grew quiet.

The doctor knocked lightly, before opening the door, entering the room, and sitting on the wheeled stool across from me. He greeted me but seemed rather solemn.

He softly said, "It's not what we thought. It's cancer."

I immediately started asking questions.

What did this mean?

What did that mean?

What was the plan?

Often in the movies, bad news is given by someone in a white coat. The camera pans to the character receiving the news. The focus of their face starts to blur as voices echo and garble, signifying the unexpected dramatic confusion...

Yeah, that didn't happen to me.

In answer to my numerous questions, the doctor gently said, "Usually, we have you come back to discuss more in detail with your spouse, because often people don't recall much after the word *cancer*."

"Well, you don't know me." I may have thought it—maybe I really said it. It doesn't matter now. I wasn't trying to be difficult. I *needed* answers.

What I found was that the pathology report was not yet complete. The mass had been measured, weighed, and examined. The report revealed poorly differentiated infiltrating ductal carcinoma (IDC), and surgical margins involved the tumor. The cancer cells were present at the edge of the tissue sample, which meant more surgery would be needed to ensure that the remaining edge and a bit more (a margin) was removed. The options were re-excision for clear margins or mastectomy (removal of the breast tissue). There would also be a sentinel node biopsy to determine whether cancer cells had spread beyond the primary tumor to the closest lymph nodes. The full pathology would take time, but once it arrived, I would know the tumor's characteristics—that means, hormone receptor status, whether the tumor was aggressive, and how different the tumor was from normal breast cells. That information would determine my treatment protocol. This appointment was in early December, and we had time to make decisions and consult an oncologist.

My husband wasn't at the appointment that day. Remember, everyone had told me they were sure it wasn't cancer. ("*Couldn't be cancer... you're too young.*") That appointment was to drop by, get some simple results, get my wound checked, and be on my way—it was supposed to be nothing. What I quickly learned was that the obligatory denials of the real possibility of cancer were too easily given. I'd totally bought into this naïve narrative. My gut reaction: I wanted to hunt down each and every person who'd bolstered my confidence and kick them square in the ass for filling my head with their bullshit. I'd rather have had a horrible possibility on the table and then feel the amazing relief of it not being real, than to be left so unprepared for my new reality.

From the minivan, I called my husband and my older sister. Neither one had realized I had the follow-up appointment that day and they had both wanted to be there. I hadn't told them—that's how sure I was that nothing bad was going to happen. I was young and from a family with no history of breast cancer—this wasn't going to happen to me! I don't recall the exact words of the conversations, but I cried. In hindsight, a phone call wasn't the best way to deliver news as my husband neared the end of the work day. My older sister picked up the call. My sniffling, clearing of throat, and tone of voice were instant clues. She cried too.

I was about to discover that saying those simple words, "I have cancer" to people is a hell of a lot easier on the phone than in person. It was lab night for me, so I drove out to school to see my instructors and, likely, revise my plans (thank goodness for the wisdom of my advisor and the flexible 15-month nursing program). Blotchy faced and clutching tissues, I arrived at my class. My instructors wanted me to reschedule my lab, but I needed to do something normal. And I didn't want to leave my partner hanging as our task was intravenous (IV) access on a patient, and student nurses practice most things on each other. So I stayed.

Knowledge is power. I got online to learn more (not something I would advise to everyone now). My husband thought I was obsessed with the computer. I justified the time in front of the screen by saying I needed to know my options and consider the numbers. Search results told me the location of that ugly jellybean was rather rare. The lower inner quadrant was the least common location for breast cancers (Lippincott). Women at my age had less than a 2% chance of being diagnosed with breast cancer (NIH SEER data). A woman's lifetime risk of breast cancer was 12%. Best case scenario, the cancer is voted off the island and is gone forever. Worst case scenario, my future involved a possible mastectomy, then possibly chemotherapy, then possibly radiation. For me, knowing the best-case and worst-case scenarios made anything in between okay with me.

Meeting the oncology doctor was a turning point. The oncologist determined the game plan after surgery. It was nearly identical to the worst-case scenario, but this time I was prepared. The tumor was estrogen receptor negative (ER-), progesterone receptor negative (PR-), HER-2 negative (HER2-), also known as triple negative breast cancer (TNBC), and rather aggressive. After more surgery for clear margins and testing the lymph nodes, there would be 6 rounds of chemotherapy (chemo). I would probably lose my hair. I might get sick. But I could probably stay in school as long as my bloodwork remained normal and I wasn't at increased risk of infection. Towards the end of chemo, I would meet a radiation oncologist for that treatment plan.

As 2003 drew to a close, the shit had hit the fan. A war had been declared inside my body. A malignant mass had been identified. That attacker was cut out with a surgeon's scalpel, and the cancer battle would continue with chemical warfare. Chemotherapy would hunt down rogue cancer cells for destruction. The last engagement would be radiation to nuke any cancer particles that tried to remain after surgery and chemo. A truce would be called when there was no evidence of disease (NED).

There's definitely a difference between knowing your shit and knowing you're in deep shit.

2

ON THE SHIT LIST

Y ou can get lost in an illness. After the initial insult, shock, and beginning the plan of care, you have to track so many things. Into an already busy, full life, suddenly your dance card is filled with numerous appointments, scans, and bloodwork, as well as planning for childcare, scheduling time off work, and paperwork for various insurance policies. And while doing all of these things, you are also trying desperately to maintain some semblance of normalcy. Everything in your life becomes a delicate balancing act.

For our family, this preparation stage involved contacting a number of people to tell them the diagnosis. They needed to know that things would be different for a while. Our finely tuned routine was going to be even more complicated since we lived a four-hour drive from any family. I took medical leave from work. We met with people at our daughter's school and our son's pre-school. Knowing our situation, they said they would work together and with us to help care for my kids. My husband's boss and coworkers encouraged him to take off whatever time was needed. My sister's family and my in-laws came to visit. I reached out to my high school friend (who had become a surgeon) for advice and asked her to share information with the others that I had cancer.

I had cancer.

Saying it over and over was exhausting, but the love and support was overwhelming. Cards, flowers, and gift baskets arrived with words of encouragement sent by family and friends all the way from Buffalo, New York, to Las Vegas, Nevada, and other points across the country.

A few busy weeks followed with more tests and procedures. I had another surgery, with the surgeon going back into the breast and taking out extra tissue for clear margins. The doctor then performed a sentinel node biopsy (SNB) to find the closest and most likely lymph node candidates to test for evidence of the cancer spreading. That was followed by a multigated acquisition scan (MUGA) to test my heart's capacity and function as a baseline before I started chemotherapy. I had a bone scan, where the technician injected a nuclear substance and then x-rayed my body to look for possible cancer in my bones (cancer would attract the nuclear material). This was followed by the placement of a Medi-Port (port), which is the implantation of a device in the upper chest just under the skin for easier access to veins; this device allows medical personnel to take blood for labs or administer intravenous (IV) fluids, avoiding a "dig" for veins in the arm. Then the chemotherapy began, purposefully poisoning my body nearly to the brink of death to hunt down and kill possible stray cancer cells. Next was radiation, which is seriously intense "tanning sessions" going straight to tender red skin without the usual healthy glow of being sun kissed.

Some people are squeamish—I get that. They can't tolerate blood, guts, needles, or pain. The details or even mention of those topics can make them upset. For those who are more sensitive, you can choose your own detailed adventure. I know a few people who probably don't want to (and may not) read the details. That's okay. My husband and I joke about me being "a beast" with all that I've had to do and tolerate. In fact, he honestly and lovingly says, "She's the toughest bitch I know."

If you want to start on my adventure with me, just turn the page and keep reading. However, if you want to skip around to the sections that interest you, check out the **Poop Scoop** (Contents) and "go" from there.

3

SCARED SHITLESS

Once you become a new member of the cancer club, your world shifts. What once seemed so incredibly important suddenly lacks any sort of urgency. Some things just don't matter when you are forced to battle for your life. And let's face it, no one chooses to join this club. I mean, why would anyone want all of their priorities to change overnight—to go from successfully managing the challenges of your life, to the next day, struggling to tread water, barely managing to keep your head above the surface in the shit creek that is now your life?

No matter how much research I'd done to prepare myself, I didn't know what was going to happen with my education, my health, and my family. There were some physical signs I was stressed. I had headaches. I got hives. I had strange abdominal pains. After being on birth control pills for nearly 14 years, I was told to stop. My body had been regulated for such a long time and suddenly it wasn't. So I needed more tests and medications for my stomach and a bladder infection.

One of the most difficult phases in dealing with cancer

happens first, waiting. The concerning mass was discovered and then you wait. You wait for appointments. You wait for tests. You wait for results. And worst, you wait for the effects of the treatment that you know are coming. Nearly a month had passed from finding the nodule in November to officially being diagnosed with breast cancer in December.

We're a society accustomed to instant gratification. Drive-thru convenience has made us less tolerant in situations that require some degree of patience. Think about fast food. You have to wait in the drive-thru lane, place an order, pull forward to pay, and wait on the bag of food. Is it really delivered to you faster than walking in? Is it as satisfying or nutritious as a homemade meal? Computers are everywhere to make life more convenient. Think about how people react when the internet is slow to load or they can't access data because of a system update or a crash. Have you had to cope without power or cable television? Those situations are minor inconveniences compared to cancer. And no one likes to wait. If you are going through as similar journey as I have, or if you have any health issue that is life-changing, my suggestion is to ask the provider when to expect the results to relieve some of the wait anxiety.

During nursing school, I'd already studied death and dying. Reading about the five stages of dealing with grief is one thing; living them is entirely different. As many of you already (and unfortunately) know, the stages include denial, anger, bargaining, depression, and acceptance (Christensen & Kockrow). I firmly believe the stages don't apply just to the loss of a loved one. A medical crisis, as well as changes in relationships or lifestyle, can be very traumatic and responding to them is a grieving process. Not everyone experiences every stage, nor do the stages proceed in an orderly fashion. There is no "right" response to a diagnosis or a "right" way to cope with treatment for the patient, their family, their friends, or coworkers. I do believe a certain respect is due to the patient and his or her family, although tact might be the more accurate terminology (see the chapter **Shitheads** for more info on this tact or the lack of it).

People make assumptions about the reasons for a cancer diagnosis. *Oh, they smoked like a chimney. Uh, look how fat they are. It's too much stress. The years of eating a crappy diet caught up with them. Must run in the family*. Why the blame game? Bad things happen for no good reason and often these assumptions are far from the truth.

You can do all the right things. Be a good person. Eat right. Exercise regularly. Not smoke. You may never know why someone got cancer. The truth is a cell somewhere in their body went haywire. If you're in the cancer club with me, don't beat yourself up over the reason why.

For fellow members of this unfortunate club, know that people will offer help. Accept it. They will say "call me if you need something!" Most of them mean it. They don't want to "bother" you, so they may not call you to check in. Then you may assume they don't care or are too busy. Assumptions like these can make a real mess. For cancer patients and the people who care about them, consider this: in the moment of "call me!" the patient says "thank you," but what well meaning friends and family don't always realize is how hard it is for an independent adult to pick up the phone and admit she needs help. If you are going through any health problem, either physical or emotional, reach out. People do care and they do want to help.

Also, get a notebook or binder to organize health information (this can be done as a team effort with family or close friends). Write down the details for appointment preparation, directions, and contacts. Write questions on paper to ask at the next appointment and take someone with you to be a second pair of ears to recall information. Any handouts from your providers can be stored in your health notebook for future reference. When you keep track of the details, it helps your caregivers intervene on your behalf when you may not feel well.

I know that's some easy advice to give, especially when you're in the thick of it. When you are sorting out the *why me, why now, what the hell am I going to do? Am I making the right choices?* When you are trusting people to take care of you, doubts can creep in. *Can I really do this? Will it hurt? Could I die?*

Again, focus on one thing at a time. Make a list of questions and concerns. The only stupid question is the one you don't ask—trust me, that's the one that will come back to bite you in the ass. Talking to the doctor, their nurse, a case manager, a social worker, or a person at the end of the 800-helpline will get you on a path to answers. Knowledge *is* power, so use the experience and expertise of others to arm yourself.

There is assistance for your emotional well-being, financial situation, and home medical equipment (among other things). Accepting help may be difficult if you've always been independent, but it is available in more places than you realize. Support groups are available for a variety of diseases, for both patients and their families. Professional counselors can prescribe methods to cope with changes in life. Think about channeling your creative side to refocus your energy in a journal, learning a craft, or resuming a hobby.

For some people, having spiritual support also helps. Years before the cancer, my approach to prayer changed. I don't recall the sermon that changed the way I pray. The gist of it was you can ask for anything and everything, but the answer isn't always yes. The answer may be "not yet," but we sometimes give up when a request isn't instantly granted. I changed from requests for specific situations to blessings for people, wisdom to assist others, patience to discern what needed to be done, and grace to cope with or understand the unknown. My hope is it will all be revealed eventually.

One way to look at life and the impact one person can make was explored in *The Five People You Meet in Heaven* by Mitch Albom. It is not a religious book about how to believe in a supreme power. It takes one man on a journey after his life ends to discover how he impacted the lives of others, even people he didn't know. The thought of how a simple act or gesture can be monumental just gives me goosebumps. So I tell my friends that despite all the shit that was generously heaped upon me, I'm going to use my powers for good to help others.

At the end of the day, we only have one life to live, so we must attempt to make the most of it. Don't doubt yourself or the decisions you make based on what information you have at the time. You are capable of amazing, extraordinary things. It's not easy to cope with challenges in life. Trying to get a grip on why things happen and what they mean takes time. Start with one task. Complete it and move onto the next task.

Once you know you've been dealt a shitty hand, just remember the game ain't over. Discard what you can. Learn to delegate to others. Allow your support people to do what they can. Take it one day at a time.

4

DO BEARS SHIT IN THE WOODS?

For details on why or how any procedure is performed, you should consult your physician, read information provided by the facility that will perform the procedure, or obtain information from a reputable website.

So what happens when you find a lumpy something in your breast? The process may differ for any one of the procedures, but I'll share my experiences with you on the radiology stuff: mammogram, ultrasound, MUGA, bone scan, positron emission scan (PET), breast magnetic resonance imaging (MRI), and ultrasound-guided biopsy.

My first step was a visit to my PCP. We reviewed my medical history and discussed the lump. She was able to feel it and suggested a baseline mammogram. Remember, I was 32 years old and mammograms usually start at middle age. Having something palpable in your breast bumps that timeline up significantly. Had I not found a lump, I would have waited for fabulous forty or nifty fifty as some studies suggest and I might not be here for you to read about my experience. More on that later.

In the simplest terms, a mammogram is an x-ray of the breast tissue while it is pressed down. That's it. Maybe you've seen cartoons or jokes flattening the breast tissue to pancakes, but that's not reality.

When you schedule a mammogram, you'll get instructions about the procedure. You'll be told where to go, when to arrive, and to hold off using lotion, underarm deodorant, or powder that morning. Don't worry about being stinky—you can apply your normal products afterward. Any of those personal products can complicate the x-ray process (it's hard to maintain a position if the tissue is slick and products can complicate the imaging process). You'll be shown to a room to change, using a cape or gown that should open to the front for the upper body.

There are screening mammograms and there are diagnostic mammograms. A screening mammogram is for people who are having their yearly study, those who have no lumps, pain, or skin changes. You show up, have imaging done, and leave. Results go to your doctor and you might get a letter in the mail.

A mammography technician will explain what to do and will position you. While you stand at the machine, the breast tissue is placed upon a tray. Then a clear plate is lowered from above to compress and hold the breast in place. You hold still for a few seconds and that angle is done.

For people with breast concerns, such as pain, palpable changes like lumps, or thickening or nipple discharge, there are diagnostic mammograms. Depending on where the lump or issue might be, several angles or views may be needed. They may have you wait while the technician consults the radiologist. They're checking to make sure all the images are technically satisfactory and that no other x-rays are needed before you leave, so you don't have to return.

The mammogram process is not as scary as cartoons make it out to be. You will not be clamped in a vice for an undetermined amount of time. Okay, there is the element of someone else seeing and manipulating your naked breasts and torso. But really, it's a relatively short process done by professionals who see hundreds, probably thousands, of breasts a year.

The technicians won't tell you if they see anything unusual on any test. They are not allowed to interpret or give a diagnosis. A radiologist has to fully review the x-rays, compare them to any previous mammograms, and determine the official findings. A report is then sent to your doctor who will tell you the results.

My results noted extremely dense tissue with a 1.4 centimeter mass and recommended further evaluation.

In her book entitled *Dr. Susan Love's Breast Book*, Dr. Love wrote, "dense breast tissue can hide a cancer, so it's sort of like looking for a polar bear in the snow."

My mammogram report also recommended an ultrasound.

An ultrasound uses sound waves to diagram structures in the body. Similar to the mammogram, you'll be told where and when to go and any details about preparing for the test. You'll get another superwoman cape or gown to change into that may be girly pink or purple (if you're lucky, it may be flowery pastels!). The technician will position you for the exam, usually reclined on a gurney or table. There will be a handheld probe with gel guided over your skin by the technician. The technician watches a computer screen for images and moves the probe around for a few minutes, pausing to type a detail or label, then repositioning a few times. Before you leave, a radiologist may briefly review your images to ensure everything is recorded.

My ultrasound results noted a 1.7 centimeter slightly irregular nodule at the 5 o'clock position of the right breast. It was not a simple cyst but a suspicious abnormality, and further evaluation with aspiration was recommended. So I went to a local surgeon for that (see **Cut the Shit**).

My cancer diagnosis prompted additional tests.

The MUGA and bone scan are radiology tests with IV contrast administered. The MUGA checked my heart function, giving a baseline reading before chemo. Some chemo drugs have the potential to damage heart function. The bone scan looked for possible spread of cancer to my bones. The x-rays picked up traces of the special IV medication in my body, and from these x-rays, a radiologist could determine whether there were any additional problems based on how the medication circulated and settled in my body.

The results of these tests showed no problems for me.

After going through the treatment trifecta (surgery, chemo, and radiation), I was monitored by my oncologist. There were follow-up appointments, lab work, and various scans. Screening and diagnostic mammograms have already been detailed, so we'll skip to PET scans.

PET scans are similar to computed tomography (CT) scans. The major difference is the preparation and contrast used. For a PET scan, a special nuclear glucose contrast material is injected into a vein. The contrast then travels through the body's circulation and is attracted to areas of increased metabolism, which could be cancer, an injury, or activity after the contrast was administered. Following preparation directions and sitting calmly during the scan are very important. The PET scan is a fasting test, so no eating after midnight or the morning of the test. Wear some comfortable clothes without any zippers, buttons, or clasps—sweats are best.

After you check in, a technician will check your blood sugar and start IV access to administer the nuclear material. No worries, you will not be transformed into a comic book hero (sorry if that was your hope for just a millisecond there). Then you sit. You can watch television (if it works in the room) or read. No knitting because that's an activity and could skew the results. Just as you might start to fall asleep, they'll knock and escort you to the imaging room, which has a CT machine, except it looks like a partial wall with a donut hole in it. You lay on your back, knees elevated on a wedge for comfort, with your arms positioned above your head. Any glasses, earrings, watches, or clothes with buttons or metal are not permitted. Without my glasses, I can't read a watch or a clock on the wall, so I couldn't tell you exactly how long it takes. The bed glides back and forth through the donut of the machine. You'll hear the spinning of gears, the tone changing with the inner movement of the scanning mechanism. I usually doze. When the whirring noises and bed motion stop, I wake up. My arms are usually tingling and numb because they started to fall asleep. My shoulders are sore too, but the rest of me is good to go. Time to eat!

A breast MRI is another specialized procedure. For women who still menstruate, it has to be timed specifically to your cycle. You'll be asked to don your superhero cape with "opening to the front please" (because there's that infinitesimal chance you aren't aware your breasts are the part being scanned that day, right?). Then you'll have an IV started. You get fancy plastic stickers to mark previous scars and the nipples (temporary removable bling).

The technician will escort you to the MRI room. There is a moveable platform bed. On my first breast MRI, my feet went toward the tube-like machine; on a more recent study at a different facility, I was head first into a rather spacious machine. You lay on your stomach with breasts hanging into cone-shaped crevices. Your arms are placed in front of you and a pillow is placed for your head to rest upon. Basically, you're doing a superman position with your breasts hanging in the cones of shame. Be careful how you put your head. I thought I'd rest my chin on the pillow and look out, but the pillow was soft and I regretted my choice as my face sunk nose-deep into it during the test. During my last MRI study, there was a special torso and head cradle, which allowed me to breathe easier, and my arms rested at my sides. The MRI machine made whirring-clanking-banging noises, which is normal. My technicians asked what music I'd like to listen to during the test—I thought that was pretty fancy. At some point, you might feel the IV contrast being administered ("you might feel warm, pressure on your bladder like you want to pee...but it'll pass..."). When the scan is done, the technicians take out the IV, you get changed and head out, and begin the wait for the results from your doctor.

Another possible test is an ultrasound-guided breast biopsy. A doctor is able to utilize ultrasound to locate a lump, note any surrounding blood vessels to avoid, and take a sample for microscopic examination. You'll change into a superhero cape, open to the front because you'll be flashing those breasts around again. A technician will have you lay on a gurney. I was awake for my procedure, so no IV sedation or access was used. The breast skin is cleaned with antiseptic. The technicians use an ultrasound probe with gel to find the mass, and then the radiologist determines how to proceed based on what is seen around the mass. Numbing medication allows the radiologist to insert a small special instrument into the skin to access the lump. I felt a bit of movement, an odd scraping sensation (not discomfort really), as the radiologist took samples. A radiology clip was placed in my breast for future location and study of the area. The instrument was then removed. Afterward, the technician held pressure, and applied Steri-strips and a dressing to the biopsy site. They gave me an ice-pack and an ace bandage to hold it in place. Done. I got dressed and went home to wait for results.

It has been a few years since I had some of these tests and procedures may have changed or may vary among facilities. There are newer techniques and updates in technology available that I did not experience. For details on tests I didn't cover, or how your physician and facility may do a procedure, consult your physicians or a reputable source.

5

CUT THE SHIT

My ultrasound results advised fine needle aspiration, so I went to a local surgeon.

The whole procedure was completed at the surgeon's office. As the name states, *it did involve a needle*. After a physical exam and short discussion, the surgeon did the procedure. First, the site was cleansed with antiseptic. Second, a bit of numbing medicine was used, and third, a small needle was inserted into the lump. The surgeon pulled back on the plunger to remove and examine any fluid from the lump that made it into the syringe, which would indicate a possible cyst. Unfortunately, there was no fluid in my lump.

We agreed to take out the lump on the same day at the doctor's office. In the procedure room, the skin was prepared with antiseptic. Some numbing medication was injected. An incision was made, and the lump was located. Within a few minutes, the mass was cut out and placed into a special container to be sent off and examined. After a few sutures, a dressing was applied. I got my bra and top back on, made an appointment to follow up, and went home. Later that evening, the numbing medicine wore off and the breast tissue was tender and sore, but it wasn't horrible pain.

A few days after the excisional biopsy, we knew we were dealing with cancer and there were possibly some cells left inside me. The choices were re-excision or mastectomy. In other words, take some more tissue to ensure clear margins (that the edge of the cancer cells was also removed) or take all the breast tissue on the right side.

It was shocking to know I had cancer, but the choice now was what to do about it. The surgeon might have removed all the cancer, but we had to make sure. Mastectomy would be a bigger surgery with a longer recovery time. The tricky thing is that even if all the breast tissue is removed, if the cancer recurs, it could just go into the chest wall.

I didn't know anyone who ever had to make this kind of decision. The re-excision (with chemo and radiation) would give me pretty much the same odds as mastectomy. Recovery time was less with re-excision. If a recurrence were to happen —and that's a big *if*—I was thinking chest wall sounded pretty bad. And I wasn't quite ready to part with my breasts. They had supplied nutrition to my infant children and, although not generously proportioned, they were mine and my husband seemed to like them. It also seemed like just the right breast went wrong. After considering our family situation and being in nursing school, I went with the breast-conserving option of re-excision.

After making the decision, we scheduled the surgery that would take place at the hospital on the same day as the sentinel node mapping.

We arrived. I changed into a surgery gown and as you'd expect, it opened to the front. During this procedure, a nuclear tracer would be injected into my right breast. The material would indicate which lymph node was the first "drain" of the lymph nodes; this was called the sentinel lymph node and needed to be removed for microscopic exam for cancer cells.

A technician and the radiologist arrived with a sealed lead tube. The contents would be injected near the original lump area. I was told, the injection "might sting a bit." *Sting a bit, my ass*! I'm usually not squeamish, but this felt worse than a mosquito's sting. Imagine if you will, a papercut or torn cuticle on your finger, applying alcohol gel, and not being able to flap your hands to dry the alcohol because it's the inside of your *breast* that's on fire. Then I was given the joyous task of massaging the breast tissue to assist circulation and drainage to the nearest lymph node.

After a short time, I was taken to radiology and I lay under the scanner. The plan: the lymph node would light up and then be marked. Then I'd go to surgery to have it removed.

I lay there for quite a while, before my surgeon was called in to see the results. The quickest lymph nodes to light up were the intermammary lymph nodes near my sternum, not the axillary lymph nodes in the armpit as one would usually expect. The problem with that is, it is difficult to access the intermammary nodes inside the chest cavity without cracking open the ribcage (which I learned afterward, and I'll explain why this is important later). So, rather than the intermammary lymph nodes that lit up the fastest, the axillary node that lit up was marked and I was taken to surgery.

In the holding area, the nurse anesthetist "pushed" some pre-op meds to relax me. They burned all the way up my arm. I said so, and I got a "sorry, sometimes that happens." *Thanks*.

When I started to wake up, I remember the nurse telling me she'd been in my shoes. She was a breast cancer survivor, so we had cancer in common, as well as nursing. She instructed me to breathe and move my feet. I joked in my drugged stupor about having a negative Homan's sign and then proceeded to ask if I had a "Smurf" boob. Huh? If you are a healthcare professional, you may be chuckling (I definitely did say and ask that). Assessing for a blood clot in the legs by having patients move their feet is normal, but not everyone knows that's what a nurse is doing. I also knew that during surgery a blue dye would be injected for visual, and a Geiger counter would be used to help find the "hot" radioactive lymph node.

A neighbor came to the hospital that day. I did not see her before or after surgery, but she somehow knew it was important to sit with my husband during the procedure. We didn't have any local family, so he was dealing with all of this alone. She jokingly said afterward that she was just being nosy, but I'm grateful for her kind heart that day.

After surgery, we discovered one of my no-no meds was Demerol. I'd heard it was evil. Someone gave me a shot in the rear; a short time later, my body gave me a lovely gift of profuse vomiting and retching. In fact, I donated my stomach contents to the porcelain gods four times in a 24-hour period. Could it have been the Lortab complicating things too? Either way, both were duly noted for future reference.

My journal, written while I went through all of this, listed post-operative details. Some entries described my husband as having the talent to be a nurse, bathing assistant, and hairdresser. Also, with the dressing site in my right arm pit, I couldn't wear deodorant. In short, it stunk. Literally.

The pathology report from this procedure was favorable. The lymph nodes taken from under my armpit showed no evidence of cancer cells. My journal entry from 1-20-2004, states, "*No nodes was good nodes.*" The rest of the breast tissue removed did not have any cancer cells either. It seemed I was Stage I, no metastasis, and triple negative. Invasive ductal carcinoma (IDC) was the most common type of breast cancer of all breast cancers.

Whoa.

Wait just a minute.

You mean there is more than one type of breast cancer?

Yep!

There are several types of breast cancer based on where the original cells went rogue. Treatment paths are based on the stage, type (place where it originated), aggressiveness, and characteristics. There are standard protocols, but not every person gets the same course of treatment.

The next procedure would be a port, which would allow easier access to my circulation for chemo. Most people don't like to be poked multiple times for an IV or for blood work. With a port, a nurse inserted a special needle into the port, then drew blood for labs or attached IV lines for chemo. There would be no digging for a vein and less chance of complications. Without a port, there was a chance that an IV site in my hand or arm could dislodge, leak out of the vein or completely "blow," allowing fluids to escape. These fluids would infuse not into my circulation, but into the tissue of my skin and muscle that could be damaged.

The port procedure was performed at the hospital. After changing into a gown and having an IV started in my arm, I was wheeled back to surgery, given anesthesia, and a new port. A pocket was made on my upper left chest. The surgeon connected the port tubing to a vein in my neck. The medical staff tested the port, stitched me closed, and put a dressing over the little bump just under my left clavicle. I woke up and went home.

There is a good reason why post-op care instructions are reviewed and given on paper. When you have surgery, you and your responsible person have to sign papers prior to sedation or anesthesia that the patient will behave, not sign any important documents, or drive until the following day when all their faculties resume normal operation. On the day of my port surgery, I had been home for three hours. We ate dinner as a family. I was wide awake and doing well, and my husband left to take our daughter to her gymnastic lesson. Our four-year-old son was home with me to relax and watch television, while the snow fell outside. My husband called to say that our four-wheel-drive sport utility vehicle (SUV) wouldn't restart for him at the gas station just a block away.

My son and I bundled up and went out to the minivan. I buckled him into his seat on the driver's side and got in the driver's seat. I was about to shift into reverse.

"Mom, the door's open," my son said.

Sure enough, I was awake but had missed an important detail, like closing the sliding door beside my child! I got out and closed the door, then drove around the block and parked. My husband used the van to jump the SUV and we all went back home.

Chemo started the next day, and the day after that, we got a new battery installed in the SUV. A word to the wise: details matter, so follow your post-op instructions.

The port would be my pal throughout treatment. Between the port access and the other injections, I had 92 "pokes" with needles from January to August 2004. The number would probably have been higher if I had not had the port, but I was still happy to have it taken out when I was done. That removal day in late August 2004 represented a freedom from illness.

The port left me with a small scar on my upper left chest that can be seen when I wear a tank top or bathing suit. Only one person has ever remarked negatively about it and they should have known better. Scars usually have stories. If someone was bold enough to ask, I was prepared to give them a fictitious tale. No one has ever inquired, but it doesn't hurt to be prepared.

6

SHIT FACED

Chemo evokes certain images in the mind. Gaunt, pale, sad faces wearing loose caps or scarves atop a bare noggin. Emaciated bodies forced to lie about without enough energy to eat. They are poor souls unable to control the direction of their stomach contents.

I don't think there is a person on Earth who looks forward to chemo. There are some who desperately want to avoid it. They weigh the odds of temporary baldness, gastrointestinal discomfort, and fatigue against the chance that a microscopic cell might grow or spread in the future. I have never been a big risk taker, and when my doctors advised chemo for the best possible outcome, I agreed.

There are a few things that can make chemo less traumatic. Ask for meds for nausea, for pain, and for upset stomach and diarrhea. Know there will be good days and not-so-good days. Report to your care team the odd things that happen: temperature, strange body pains, unusual headaches, sinus drainage, sore throat, cough, tender teeth and gums, rashes, bruising, bleeding, gynecological changes, even insomnia. All of these symptoms can signal to your doctor to treat an issue that could complicate your health. Have some people who can back you up with childcare, meals, and even transportation. Know your friendly foods (crackers, oatmeal, cream of wheat, applesauce) and have some on hand. Keep in mind, the cancer and chemo experience is different for everyone.

The treatment plan for my breast cancer was six rounds of chemo. The staff would pre-medicate me with anti-nausea meds. The Ativan, Anzemet, and Decadron cocktail came thru my IV before they administered the FEC regimen (5-fu, Epirubicin, Cytoxan). The day after my new port was implanted, my husband drove me to my first round of chemo. We checked in and were assigned a recliner in the infusion room. Even though it was a group atmosphere, the other people there for treatment kept to themselves, supervised by the staff. The nurses used a special needle to access my port and started the infusion.

I'd been told that drinking a cold drink during infusion would help prevent mouth sores later. That seemed like a good idea, until that strawberry slushy gave me a strange gurgle-swooshy belly that turned into explosive diarrhea. So there I was, tethered to a beeping IV pump on a pole, with a nurse tap-tap-tapping at the bathroom door, "Are you ok?" Yes. And no. With no outlet in the restroom, the beeping continued until my body allowed me to return to my assigned seat. I still feel badly about the entire infusion room full of patients just outside the bathroom overhearing the episode and for the next person who had to go in there. The entire chemo appointment lasted a few hours. Then we went home. And that was my chemo routine.

The chemo circulated through my body. Its job was targeting rapidly dividing cells and destroying them, but chemo doesn't differentiate between friend (hair, gastrointestinal track, and some blood cells) and foe (cancer). Chemo patients lose their hair, their lunch, their bowels, their appetite—that's how chemo works.

There are many predictable responses to chemotherapy. With different cancers, different chemo regimens, different responses to treatment, not everybody has the same issues. As the chemo did its job, my body responded. Red-colored urine was expected with one of my drugs. The medical staff encouraged me to drink plenty of fluids and flush the toilet twice. Nausea was possible. Strong smells were definitely a problem for me (cooked bacon, floor waxing at a clinical facility, some anonymous woman's strong perfume in public). I learned to pre-medicate or leave an area to avoid vomiting. Constipation and the foul opposite of it, diarrhea, were also possible (stress can shut you down or speed you up). Hair loss was possible, so I tried to control that by getting mine cut shorter in stages. Low blood cell counts often complicated, even delayed, treatment until my issues were solved.

Blood cells in the body don't have a significantly long life-span and are constantly in production. When certain types of blood cells die off without being replaced, there are signs and symptoms that go along with each cell type. Low red blood cell counts make a person tired and lethargic. Low platelet count manifests with bruising and bleeding easily. Having low white blood cell counts open a person up to the possibility of dangerous infections.

White blood cells are the lookout soldiers of the body. They are on guard to fend off foreign invaders (like viruses and bacteria), engulfing and destroying enemies in our bodies. When the troops are low in number, bacteria flourish, and the body can't mount a proper defense. If the person doesn't get medical attention (being prescribed medications like antibiotics), the body will be overwhelmed by massive infection and will eventually start to shut itself down, possibly resulting in death.

When a chemotherapy patient has a low white count, precautions are needed to prevent complications from potential infection. Proper handwashing and staying away from public places/crowds or people with known infections are key. A doctor will not immunize/vaccinate a chemo patient with a live virus, and the patient needs to stay away from people who have recently had shots with a live virus (like young children receive regularly with well-child visit immunizations). Fresh fruits and vegetables can harbor bacteria, so they need to be fully cooked before eating. Peeling the fruit or vegetable skin can contaminate the inner material of the produce. Leftovers from the refrigerator need to be reheated to a boiling point, which isn't possible in the microwave. Gifts of plants or flowers can bring unusual bacteria into the home and from there, contact with the patient. I'm not being paranoid. The dangers are real. Something you may not ordinarily think about could lead to a serious hospitalization or worse for someone with a compromised immune system.

There are medication injections that can kick start the white cell defense system. You've probably seen the advertisements on television for the injections that warn "mild to moderate bone pain." My white cell count tanked, and I had to have the injections. The shot itself was administered into the fatty tissue of the lower abdomen and it burned a little. In the following few days, I experienced pain in my femurs, hip carriage, sternum, and back. It was so debilitating, my husband asked friends from church (thanks B & J!) to drive me to get the shots for my own safety. He was concerned pain might impair my ability to steer or brake in an emergency during the 30-minute drive to the clinic.

I often wonder whether the copywriters for the ads have ever used the medication. If that were the case, the ad might more accurately be revised to include, "potential to make you creak, stoop, and not want to breathe due to great and unusual pain, so make sure you ask for an opioid pain reliever just in case."

Ever had sunburn on your scalp? A week after my first infusion, my scalp was tender and itchy like that sunburn feeling. The hair started to loosen and a few strands would come out when I ran my hands through it. I could shake my head over the bathtub and it would release more strands. After a few days of massive shedding, we went to the barber. I got a shave like Demi Moore in *GI Jane*.

When my husband asked how much, the barber replied, "No charge."

We thanked him and left. Then I lost it. Yes, I'd lost my hair, but that was not what made me bawl. It was the entire unfair mess that cancer had given me. (See **My Shit Don't Stink** for further details.)

Your head gets cold without hair. My choice to deal with my newfound baldness was not wigs or their proper medical terminology, hair prosthesis—I was too afraid the wig would fall off in front of a patient during my clinical school days. I figured it was better to be honest about my follicular impairment, and I rocked the do-rags and hats. On non-school days, I must have looked like such a badass with my do-rags and hoop earrings! Okay, maybe I *thought* I looked like a badass even though most of my head wraps were pink or patterns (hardly a menacing vision). I also lacked physically imposing muscles or a burly motorcycle.

My lack of hair was challenging at times. You don't really worry about your hair matching your outfit, but a do-rag? It requires a bit of thought. However, having no hair made getting ready for the day quicker without having to shampoo, blow-dry, and style. And I also didn't have to shave my legs. The hair was absent everywhere eventually—head, eyebrows, eyelashes, arms, and down there.

You don't think about the little hairs in your nose much of

the time, do you? They filter what goes in and slow down what goes out. After those hairs have vacated, if you feel like you have a runny nose, your sinus drainage is already leaking onto your top lip or dripped down to your chin (not the sexist feeling ever).

(FYI- yes, the hair goes away, but a few weeks after I finished chemo, the hair on my head sprouted and looked like duck fuzz. As it grew longer, the texture and color changed to a sleek, peppery, edgy look. A few months later, my own color and curls returned. Some people have other changes in texture and color when their hair comes back after chemo.)

Chemo continued to give me a few challenges, including headaches, green chunks of goop from my nose, and low-grade temperatures, all indicating sinus infections. Antibiotics were prescribed. A magic mouthwash helped for sensitive teeth, achy gums, tender mouth, and throat soreness. Nosebleeds happened just when blowing my nose. My menstrual cycle stopped (BONUS!!!). Loss of appetite due to metallic taste changes, nausea, and vomiting occurred with strange regularity in the chemo cycle.

If it wasn't coming out the top, it was surprising me at the other end. One time, I didn't make it to the restroom in public. In my defense, my colon gave very little warning. At 32 years old, I had diarrhea pooped myself. I ripped off my underwear and deposited them in the ladies' room sanitary disposal. That's actually an oxymoron, isn't it? Sanitary disposal—what goes in there really isn't sanitary, right? I went home commando.

Then a strange itchy area popped up, angry and red, on my right side.

SHINGLES!

At times, it's difficult to see what's going on with yourself. At one point, a friend called to check on me. I told her I'd been sick to my stomach on and off for five days, achy all over, and just couldn't keep anything down. She said I probably needed IV fluids, and told me to call my doctor. We dropped the kids off with friends and went in for a checkup. After three liters of fluid with potassium and some steroids, I felt a whole lot better!

Nursing school continued with clinical days scheduled around my chemo infusions. I missed only one clinical day due to illness. To make a deadline one month, I had to take a test I didn't feel prepared for and still passed, but not with my usual grade. Tink and Bubba kept to their school and activities schedule. My husband worked but took days off for my treatments.

Being an advocate for yourself is a must. When you leave a message but people don't call back, don't assume it's because your issue is not really a problem. Sometimes people get busy—they don't understand how shitty you feel because they've never experienced how awful chemo is or they just suck at their jobs. Call again or go in to be seen. I had to show up without an appointment and relay to my doctor in person that her staff had not addressed my calls. She was disappointed to learn of my difficulty and attributed it to a new staff member without oncology experience, who didn't know my particular case history. Don't settle. Ever. If you just can't be that bold, have someone be your muscle. They can be the tough guy, the bad cop, the bitch, because sometimes they have to be. This is your life! That's pretty flippin' important right?!

The six rounds of chemo finished in May 2004. My chemo graduation day was kind of a downer. My last infusion was delayed due to low blood counts, and I was at a different facility with none of the usual patients or staff. If I hadn't said it was my last, I'm not sure I would have received my graduation certificate.

One week after my last round of chemo, I had a really

strange day. I had a hard time sleeping and woke thinking of all the odd events leading up to my diagnosis. I made my way to the city for a Procrit shot to bring up my blood counts and then out to school to do some work in class. I grabbed some lunch with two friends and came back to the lab room. There were a few students watching one of the assigned videos called *The Doctor*. I had viewed it already and knew what was about to happen in the movie—I had to excuse myself from the room before I lost it. I fled to the restroom and ran into Mrs. F (our director of nursing).

We had a brief exchange and I almost used the word epiphany, but instead asked her, "Have you ever had a true moment of clarity?"

She responded, "An epiphany?"

So I started telling her the details of my night awake. Knowing two women with benign breast issues prior to my cancer and the timing of certain modules in the program that pertained to cancer were remarkable. The pain conference we attended before my lump and diagnosis included breast cancer survivors. The movie playing in lab that day was what tied it all together for me. The extraordinary events that fore-shadowed my own cancer diagnosis, in retrospect, somehow softened the blow to my own mortality. All the bizarre devel-opments in less than 12 hours were an epiphany! Yes, cancer was shitty, but I was still alive for a purpose yet to be determined.

I felt compelled to contact someone from the pain conference to thank them for the timely presentation. Turns out, Mrs. F had just received something from them! I didn't run into her often, so seeing her that day was yet another wonder to add to my day. I did send a letter to the pain conference organizer on how beneficial it was for me.

I had a follow-up appointment with the oncologist a few weeks after my last chemo. I asked what my official stage was.

What I understood was it was Stage I, but what about those lymph nodes that lit up in the middle of my chest, before the ones in my armpit? The doctor replied that it was possible those could have had cancerous cells and if they did, I would have been a Stage III. But we'd never know for sure about those lymph nodes in my chest. Since it wasn't easy to biopsy them without cracking open the chest, we'd treated systemically with chemo and would proceed with radiation.

So on paper, I was officially Stage I, which was good. Statistics were in my favor for Stage I. In the grand scheme of things, *possibly* Stage III was not good. Breast cancer stages range from I to IV. Stage I is smaller than an inch and well contained. The stages increase in number with regard to the size of the tumor and how far cancer cells have migrated from the site of origin. Stage IV is cancer with metastasis to other organs or bones outside the original site, possibly or eventually terminal when it stops responding to treatment. On the upside, my chemo was finally done and I was moving on to the next phase of treatment.

7

HOT SHIT

R adiation (rads) commenced after the end of chemo. The radiation oncologist's office and adjacent treatment center were located in what would be considered the basement of the building. The doctor met with my husband and me to discuss the plan. I would have some testing and marking done to know where and how to treat the right breast area. Because I had the internal mammary chain (area along the middle of my chest) of lymph nodes light up before the axillary (underarm) lymph nodes, the doctor would treat that area as well.

The testing process was called simulation. A CT scan would map my organs, and that map would help guide the depth of treatment and avoid damaging parts of my body that didn't need radiation. They drew lines with a black Sharpie from my neck down my sternum, across the top and bottom of the right breast, as well as my side to armpit, marking the radiation fields. I got my first tattoos, which permanently marked the edges of the radiation field. Don't freak out—they were no bigger than the head of a pin. The medical staff give you tats to show where you had treatment to avoid radiation of that area in the future.

Radiation started in June 2004 and would last into July. There would be 33 total treatment days. That meant 33 trips to the city (30-40 minutes one way) that took longer than the actual treatments (less than 20 minutes once I was on the table).

Since I had black marker going straight up the middle of my chest to the base of my throat, I started wearing mock-neck tops in public, so people wouldn't see or ask about the markings. Mock-neck tops in Oklahoma during June and July, you say? Yes, I was definitely *hot*, and I don't mean *sexy* hot.

Monday through Friday, I had appointments in the late afternoon, which allowed me to continue school and clinical days. I would arrive and change into a gown that (say it with me now) opened in the front (as always, right?) for my "tanning session." When I was called into the treatment room, I climbed up on the table. The staff positioned me under a machine that looked like an x-ray machine. They used specially made casts to point the radiation to certain areas while I lay there, gown open and pesky breast waiting to be nuked. They then changed the machine's position to treat three different field angles and then I was done.

After two weeks of trips to Tulsa for treatments, I felt a small knot just below my right nipple. The doctor checked with ultrasound but couldn't identify a mass, so I was sent to my surgeon. He removed the mass and sent it off to pathology. It was about the size of a pea and showed some dye from my surgery months before. Three days later, we received pathology results showing no malignancy. So my radiation treatments continued.

I experienced some reddened areas under my breast, arm, and along my sternum. Special ointments helped ease the tenderness. The skin soon peeled, and I was exhausted.

I continued to see the radiation oncologist for my mammograms. This medical professional was the person who eventually said something about my port scar.

The doctor pointed out that my scar was "unsightly."

Who did your surgery? I'm sure they can fix that.

The scar is on my upper left chest. It was not visible unless wearing a bathing suit or strapless dress. That was the last I saw of that doctor. The flippant remark made me angry that after all I'd been through, my scar was the most remarkable thing that needed to be discussed. It also felt like an attack on my surgeon's abilities. You know, the doctor whom I trusted first in my cancer experience?!? Enough was enough. I decided that day to stick with just my medical oncologist (chemo doctor) for further follow-ups and mammograms.

8

NO SHIT

So what do you do when all the treatment is done? You "graduate" and are in a sort of limbo or purgatory. Just as a young bird is pushed out of the nest, you are expected to fly out on your own with just a little diploma, maybe a celebratory bell ring, and then good luck! You're told the cancer seems to be gone. There is no evidence of disease. Maybe you're told that you're "in remission." It's really hard to find someone to say, "You're cured!" They can't promise it's gone forever and won't come back.

There you are trying to get back to living life, doing the work, family, and education routine, but it's not quite like before cancer. Each new or weird symptom makes you pause and think, what's that now? For patients previously diagnosed with cancer, the surveillance routine consists of blood tests, radiology films or scans, and periodic appointments to check for symptoms of anything unusual going on in the body.

There were check-ups every few months. Mentally gearing up to go to the facility, physically expose yourself, and wait for results was emotionally draining. I think as health care gets more advanced with electronic medical records, the process should become easier. But almost every time I showed up, there were the same forms that want your medical history of diagnosis and surgeries. Really? Again? Don't you have my file somewhere that I could just add to? It's just a suggestion from little ol' me that might expedite the process.

One time, I had a mammogram and follow-up appointment scheduled. When I arrived, they told me at radiology and the doctor's office, "I'm sorry, we don't have you listed." WHAT? You think I would pull this date out of my ass and come down here to get squished because I'm bored and it's the best thing I could think to do on a rainy day? I later found out that many "scheduled" patients didn't show, and those who showed up, "didn't have appointments." It's certainly strange in this computer age where computers are *never* wrong.

In February 2010, I found a strange area. It was a rough, reddened, but tender, dry patch on my upper left breast. It was not an area that was irritated by a bra strap since it was close to the areola. I put some moisturizer on it for a few days. Then I called my PCP and tried more moisturizer as advised. I had a mammogram that noted nothing unusual. Two weeks later, the oncologist looked at the weird area and ordered an MRI. The MRI result suggested an ultrasound because of calcification noted. Then at the ultrasound, the radiologist suggested an ultrasound-guided biopsy of a suspicious area. I am dismissed with a flippant, "Okay, we're done here. See you soon."

No joke. At that point, I'd done more research. The "sore" could have been a cutaneous manifestation of IDC. Paget's disease of the breast often presents as nipple irregularity and then IDC. The "rapid washout" noted in the MRI results often happens when a cancer is triple negative, like my cancer had been—*shit*.

Once again, two other people I knew revealed recent breast issues. Coincidence? It certainly felt like God was tapping me on the head again, saying, "Hello, wake up and take action, sister!"

I'd had the cancer experience already—been there, done that. If I had to, I'd do it again, but all the delays and timing of tests were a bit odd. My husband even mentioned that it felt kind of like a conspiracy. I felt really bad for him. It can't be easy. I knew a whole lot more about breast cancer than he did, but I didn't want to scare the shit out of him. He'd had a lot going on at work and really didn't need the additional stress.

Up to finding the new concern, I didn't think a lot about the whole cancer thing, but after finding it, I didn't want to seem like it was the only thing I could focus/talk about either. I wasn't depressed. Concerned? Yes, but I didn't have a choice about being down because that's contagious. I was actually mad—mad at everyone who told me, "It's probably nothing." What I really wanted was to kick each of their asses and yell, "DON'T TRY TO PLACATE ME! I KNOW HOW THIS SHIT WORKS!"

Twelve days later, I had the biopsy with the flippant "Okay, we're done here" radiologist. The doctor and technician talked amongst themselves above me, as if I weren't fully awake and present for the procedure. The next day, I received the results at the radiology center from the radiology tech, *not* the radiologist. Benign. The tech was surprised when I said I thought it was cancer. Had she seriously not dealt with any previous cancer patients to sense the anxiety?

By then, I'd had the strange patch for six weeks. My surgeon agreed to investigate with a biopsy and removed the entire patch of skin. Benign. Thank God. Weeks of worry were finally resolved.

9

SHIT OUT OF LUCK

W e had gotten back to living life. We had family trips, vacations, got together with friends, worked, and watched the kids at sports and music events. I'd been seeing someone for checkups at least every six months since my diagnosis in 2003. My oncologist suggested in October 2010 that it was time to go to yearly visits. Things were stable. Such a relief! I'd had no recurrence, just a few concerns that had been addressed and ruled out.

From that October to January 2011, I had three clinical breast exams during regular doctor appointments. First the oncologist, then in December my PCP, and finally in January, I went to see my gynecologist. No lumps or bumps were detected.

In February 2011, I got sick. It was so bad with abnormal bowel movements and rectal bleeding that I went to the emergency room. They advised a visit to my general surgeon and to schedule a colonoscopy. Though there were no further questionable stools after the ER visit, we proceeded with the test.

Colonoscopy preparation is the toughest part of the

entire colonoscopy experience. The prep will vary from doctor to doctor. Usually, it involves ingesting some small but powerful pills and strange tasting liquid to quickly evacuate the bowels on the day before the exam. After starting the prep, do not plan to go out. Do not plan to eat dinner or anything except what the doctor allows, clear liquids. Expect to spend some quality time in the bathroom. Buy some wet wipes or baby wipes for your bottom, because before too long, even the softest toilet paper feels like sandpaper on your poor bum.

If you're lucky, you probably won't remember much of the procedure. You sign in, change into a gown open to the back (well, they are checking your colon and that is in the back), and then they start an IV site. You are positioned on your side on a gurney, wearing oxygen tubing in your nose and wires that connect you to a monitor for your heart rate and rhythm. Then a nurse will give you some medicine in your IV. They call it light sedation, because you are awake enough to respond to questions if needed but won't remember much of anything due to the medicine. After the procedure, you'll expel extra gas from the procedure since air is used to inflate the colon for inspection. Some of the air gets trapped and it stays behind (Ha! That's funny "shit talk" there!) and exits later. Don't be surprised if some pretty loud and funny eruptions occur, even if you are not usually a person who farts. This might be something you do or do not remember later. The medical staff will assist you in getting dressed. Your ride pulls up with the car and you go home to rest. The follow-up appointment was already scheduled for the following week to discuss the procedure results.

Two days before my appointment with the surgeon to discuss the colonoscopy, I was getting ready for bed. Sometimes when you take off your bra, it's a relief to have that pressure off. You might rub where the band and straps were.

My left hand glanced over an area just to the left and below my areola on the right breast.

Wait, what?

I stopped, felt it again.

Then I grabbed my husband's hand and made him feel it. His reaction confirmed my immediate fear. This was new and different.

The follow-up appointment with the surgeon was on Thursday. I'd get the colonoscopy results, which for some reason I wasn't really worried about now. There had been a polyp removed and a biopsy of an irritated area, but that didn't worry me.

The doctor came into the exam on Thursday afternoon and said it was a *good news* day, no signs of cancer in the colonoscopy. Good news indeed, but then I had to rain on the parade.

I think the doctor may have sensed something else was going on when we showed up. I told him about finding the lump just two nights before. The doctor handed me a cape and left the room so I could change for an exam. This lump was like a small grape, tender to touch, but not moving like a cyst would. The needle aspiration didn't tell anything other than no liquid could be drawn out of the mass. The office scheduled a mammogram and ultrasound for the next day.

This doctor's office had known me for seven years. They had been a great source of support and encouragement. They had to tell me about the cancer seven years ago. They got my concerns addressed about a lump that occurred during radiation. I pestered them about removing my port when I was "done" with it. The staff had come to my graduation from LPN school. They supported me when an odd patch of skin on the left breast prompted a breast MRI and then ultrasound-guided biopsy just the year before. I'd started out as a patient, but had developed a professional relationship and friendship with these exceptional people.

The investigation cycle began.

The mammogram said dense breasts, but did not identify the palpable mass.

An ultrasound suggested a biopsy, given my history of breast cancer.

The following Monday, the lump was removed at the doctor's office. When it had been taken out, I saw it sitting on the procedure tray. It was beige, smooth, and round. I asked to glove up, so I could feel it. It was hard, unyielding to even slight pressure of my fingers. The doctor sent it off to pathology.

By Thursday, we knew it was cancer. Strange thing to note was the date, it had the same numbers but in a different combination than my first diagnosis (12/11/2003 compared to 3/2/2011).

Life was about to change again. I wasn't innocent about the things that were going to occur. Having cancer once sucks, but having it a second time is exceptionally shitty. What's the phrase? Once bitten, twice shy? Having been through the experience, you know how hard it can be for the second round.

There would be more tests.

My next surgery would be a simple (rather than radical) right breast mastectomy. The mass had developed on the same side that had been cut, poisoned, and roasted previously, but this had been a new and different tumor. Pathology said it was slightly estrogen receptor positive (7%). To decrease my chance of it occurring on the left breast in the future, I wanted a prophylactic left mastectomy if insurance would allow. A great deal of thought goes into separating yourself from your boobs. I just wanted to cut my risk as much as possible, so we also discussed a possible hysterectomy (removal of uterus and the ovaries).

My oncologist wanted a PET scan and genetic testing.

My surgeon wanted to investigate my history of lower abdomen pain and sent me for an ultrasound.

Both doctors advised a visit with a plastic surgeon before my mastectomy.

Journal entry 3-5-2011: *Have read about reconstruction. That's some scary shit. So you can get some implants that won't last forever, or pull some muscle from your tummy, back or ass to make a breast mound. Sounds like a whole lot of pain I just don't want to deal with right now.*

We all decided that breast reconstruction would be delayed until after the mastectomy, hysterectomy, and completion of chemo.

I broke the news to my family, friends, and coworkers. I would have to be off work for some time between the surgeries and chemo treatments.

At work, I was walking down the hall with my bestie there and said I'd had my follow-up and the findings were cancer. I don't recall her exact words, but I do remember how her eyes welled up and she just hugged me tight.

My husband shared the news with someone who'd witnessed the previous treatment and knew this wasn't my first rodeo. My father-in-law's reply was an emotional and justified, "F---. F---. F---, f---, f---!"

In one group text to my friends, I explained, "So, at this point I'm just waiting like a plane to land and find a gate in an unknown land, where I'm going to have to learn a new language, the customs and all that shit."

My friend responded, "... I'd add to it that you didn't choose to travel here. So not only were you forced to leave your homeland, but now you have to acclimate to a place you never intended to visit. It isn't fair."

My daughter clearly remembers the conversation in the car. She was 16 years old. We'd had a few heated discussions in the weeks prior about stunts in her dance routines that were dangerous. I was concerned about the dance stuff, but also about the cancer. She thought I was upset with her about dance and I admitted it wasn't entirely dance that had been bothering me. There was another lump. It was cancer again. She was quiet. To lighten the moment, I complained that I'd just spent $80 on my recent haircut and color that would just be wasted. That's what she remembers—not crying, but coping by laughing. We held off telling my 11-year-old son until the weekend, so he would have time to adjust to the news.

Journal entry 3-13-2011: ... *Can't talk about it but was I having premonitions of all this?... Pondering it could make you crazy really. Am I just that lucky to have 2 tumors appear in the 5% quadrant with a chance of second primary being less than 20%? Is this tumor way different? Is it the work of BRCA mutation? So much that's rare or uncommon going on. Why? I have no idea. I want to say I'm strong enough to do this again but keep waking up to the same scars, the same faint pain on the right, so it's not a bad dream.*

10

UP SHIT CREEK WITHOUT A PADDLE

My bilateral mastectomy was approved and scheduled. We arrived at the outpatient area and met up with my bestie. She came to see me before going down to work in our unit for the day. Working in a small community hospital has benefits. People know you and take care of you. My case was unusual for all of us since it was a second cancer in a 39-year-old coworker.

The surgery went well, but my recovery had complications. One problem was I couldn't urinate and there was plenty of liquid in my bladder according to a scanner, so I had to have a urinary catheter put in place temporarily. The IV site in my left arm infiltrated (fluid leaked outside of the vein and caused swelling under my skin) overnight. The pain from the IV site inside my elbow crease hurt more than the mastectomy at times. The staff encouraged me to walk, reminded me to use caution with range of motion and weight restriction, as well as checked to make sure I was as comfortable as possible and had everything I needed within reach when resting.

The next day, my surgeon said he'd consulted with my

gynecologist and oncologist. There was no sign of cancer anywhere else but the breast, which meant I was considered Stage I again. After reviewing my pelvic ultrasound results and taking into account that my cancer was estrogen receptor positive this time, the doctors advised a hysterectomy. That surgery would be scheduled in a few weeks. They could coordinate the operating schedule, so my port could also be placed while I was under anesthesia.

My husband took me home after discharge and I learned to sleep in a semi-reclined cocoon on the couch. Friends and family prayed, called, and texted. My poor husband joked about developing callouses on his thumbs from texting with everyone about me before, during, and after surgery. I posted cryptic updates on Facebook so that only the people who knew my situation would know what they meant. The recovery pain wasn't horrible even though I had drains for five days.

The drains looked like clear grenades attached to tubing that entered into my skin just under my armpits. The tubing coiled under my skin where the breast tissue had been removed. The drains would remove fluid that accumulated in the space where my breasts had been. If left unattended, fluid buildup could lead to clots or infection. Several times daily, the drains were uncapped, tipped to empty the liquid contents, re-squished, and recapped to resume their job suctioning off the excess fluid. The drains' sutures and suction felt like little monkeys pinching the inside of my arm pits. I was told to limit my activity, no lifting, no housework, no driving. As my recovery progressed, so did my range of motion in my arms and shoulders.

I'd thought about uterine ablation or having a hysterectomy a few months before due to heavy menstrual flow and severe cramps, but hadn't made a final decision. It seemed the cancer had done that for me. You gotta do what you gotta do.

At a visit before surgery, my gynecologist suggested starting a medication that might be helpful, given all the stress with another breast cancer diagnosis and the major surgeries. She explained and I completely understood that Celexa can be a brief or long-term treatment worth trying. Okay. I started it two days prior to my hysterectomy, hoping to make the hormone transition easier.

Just a month after my double mastectomy, I had an abdominal hysterectomy and a new port placed in my upper right chest. My breast cancer was not a result of genetics, but since it was ER+, getting rid of the source of estrogen was important. My gynecologist discovered some pretty gnarly endometriosis when she opened me up. My left ovary was really hesitant to leave its cozy home and was a bit of trouble to remove. My surgery was on a Friday, and I went home on Easter Sunday.

Abdominal surgery was difficult. You don't realize how much you utilize those muscles until you shouldn't use them. Again, I suffered some complications. For one thing, my weight was up eleven pounds from admission to discharge home.

Text message to friends 4-26-2011: *So I'm 4 days into menopause and believe I have my faculties back. It was weird, I may have sounded normal Friday, Saturday and Sunday- but I don't remember much thanks to the lovely meds I was on...Took a water pill and lost five pounds today. Had to buy some new undies to fit my arse and belly as I heal.*

In my post-op haze, I neglected to realize that the oral antibiotic I was prescribed to take home was in the family of a medication I had an allergic reaction to. Within a week, I was in the emergency room with a temperature and urinary tract infection, and had to start taking a new antibiotic. Within 24 hours of taking the new antibiotic, I gained a lacy rash and started feeling drunk, dizzy, and hot. Maybe hives or heat rash from hot flashes? The itching was so bad I was balling my fists to not scratch myself and shaking my limbs to get some relief. Basically, I was allergic to this medication too, so I stopped it and the Celexa I had started prior to the hysterectomy. Better safe than sorry and, emotionally, I was doing okay. Benadryl was my bestie, since it helped with the itching and sleep over the next few days.

In a short amount of time, I'd be getting chemo again. One of my tasks to prepare was to get my ears re-pierced so could wear some big ass hoops with do-rags. So I drove down to the local department chain store and picked out my posts. The jewelry counter attendant gathered her supplies, marked my ears, and then paused.

She asked if I was sure I wanted my ears pierced. I replied yes. She then asked if she should call someone over to help hold me up, because she'd had people who just couldn't tolerate it and passed out. I assured her that I would be just fine. (After all, what were three holes in my ears compared to the three surgical sites I'd had in the previous weeks?) And voila, I had my ears pierced and at the ready for those hoops.

Two good friends had gifted some hand-knit shawls to me. They were an inspiration to take up knitting to pass the time, be productive, and think about other people. Having that creative outlet was good for me and pretty low cost since I learned a lot from YouTube.

One day, we went out to eat at a local bar-b-que restaurant. They made good food and I love their sweet tea. From our booth, I could see a family at the front corner table. They had a baby with them who started to fuss. The young mother picked up the infant. She covered the baby and her chest with a blanket and started to nurse.

Tears welled in my eyes.

It was a sad moment for me when I fully realized that I would have no more babies, no more nursing, no more breasts because of cancer. I briefly left the table to compose myself in the restroom. For the most part, I hold it together really well, but seeing that simple interaction made my heart ache.

At the end of May 2011, intermittent abdominal sensations turned into horrible stabbing pains. They were so intense that my husband came home from work to take me to the emergency room. They tested my urine. They accessed my port for blood and gave me some IV medications. My husband noticed, after we got settled, that the nurse had dressed the access site, but had clamped not capped the catheter pigtail to my port. Even though there was a clamp, that port with an uncapped IV line provided direct access for air and any floating bacteria to my blood stream and heart. We brought the concern to the staff's attention and they promptly corrected it. The ER doctor told me the pain was most likely gastritis and advised follow-up with a gastrointestinal physician.

My general surgeon suggested a look at my stomach to see whether any irritation, infection, or ulcers were to blame for my pain. The study found no issues. Perhaps, it was a virus, small bowel obstruction, or adhesions.

I wasn't looking forward to chemo. It began five weeks after my hysterectomy in June 2011. This time, the chemo regimen would be premedication with Aloxi, Ativan, Decadron, Benadryl, and Zantac. Then they would give me Taxotere and Carboplatin. My husband would drive me to a facility in the city for my infusions. The day after, I would be given a shot of Neulasta to prevent my blood counts from falling too much.

After reading the educational sheets about the main chemo drugs and the possible side effects, I dreaded what was about to start. I knew about the basics from my chemo experience in 2004. This stuff also had the potential to cause fluid retention, kidney or liver function problems, hearing changes, seizures, numbness or tingling in the hands and feet, and color change and/or falling off of my fingernails and toenails.

As in the past, I journaled my experiences, symptoms, and reactions for better recall. It helped with what to expect and when it would occur in the cycle.

Nausea.

Vomiting.

Red neck and face.

Insomnia.

Constipation.

Diarrhea.

Metallic taste.

Bone pain.

Itchy sunburned scalp.

My hair started falling out and I went to my hairdresser, who shaved it for free. She said I had a beautiful head. That was a compliment considering the number of heads in different lengths and shades of hair she'd seen.

Then I experienced a new symptom that was really embarrassing—gas so horrible even the dog got up and walked away from me. I named those days "DFD" for the death farts and diarrhea that could gag a maggot.

Throat and mouth pain.

Palms of hands and soles of feet became red and tender.

Hot flashes.

For almost every symptom, there was a medicine or remedy. Then the next cycle of chemo would begin again.

Blog post 6-25-2011: *I have to share a blurb from the past few days, 'cause I really had a good time chatting, check it out. You know who you are and I shall not name you...*

Friend: Wearing pink BTW

Me: Good Girl :) waiting on the dr to see me then we hit the lounge for cocktails.

Friend: You make that sound so festive.

Me: and fun! There's "waitresses," recliners, people mingling, hors d'oeuvers, some good drugs...

Friend: U r a kook.

Me: In the lounge over in the corner...Some funny $hit people talk about. Literally. And other strange topics.

Friend: Is there a saxophonist? Dim lights? Maybe a little jazzy blues to go with your cocktail? Is that so much to ask?

Me: not too dim. No one smoking though. Weird. It's cool in here. Glad I wore pants and added a sweater as a backup. Cause you know sometimes I don't year pants...

Friend: Hahahaha. Yeah, u're like that!

Me: Wear! Damn predictive text.

The chemo was tough. It's odd how we tend to censor the actual extent of an experience as a courtesy to others. We're raised to be proper, to not discuss certain things or bother people with our troubles. I've learned since then, that this editing process doesn't really benefit a cancer patient. It diminishes the patient's feelings, cultivates their fear, and minimizes the extent of their many losses.

From journaling July 2011: *Yesterday would've been a perfect example of the concept I need to explain. It was my 5th day after chemo. I went to bed the night before with severe bone pain in my legs. The pain became intense after being achy all day. I laid down in bed with a hot pack on my knees, trying to find a position to just rest and allow my body to relax. It was a night of tossing and turning. I woke on day 5 at 7:38am. It was picture day for the dance calendar. My daughter was up, barely, and getting into the shower. That left 17 minutes for [my son] and me to get out the door too. We did it somehow. I showered, quick, not having any hair can be a perk at times. Threw on some clothes and we left.*

We were up to the memorial [photo shoot] by 8:20am. Saw a few people who remarked how good I looked and they liked my scarf. Pleasant smiles, picture done and we were on the way home. Too tired to mingle or do drive thru for drinks, just wanted to be home. So I shed my costume when I got home. Comfort over fashion. Grey Capri pants, tank top and a white do-rag. So tired. Physically drained. Nausea coming and going. Awful metal taste lingering. Mentally unable to shut off. It's exhausting. I used to work 16 hour shifts and get up the next day to take care of the house, kids or school. Now I'm lucky if a shower doesn't wear me out. It was only day 5 after chemo and it'll get better before it gets worse again. That's just the thing- I know it will.

Since March 22nd, I've made an effort. It's been an effort to get out of bed without crying, take a shower without crying and if I can pull that off, I can get on with my day. There have been losses- my health, my boobs, my uterus and ovaries. My self-image, my confidence to trust my instincts and my body... Personally, I think I've done well. But there are many reasons.

I think I've been conditioned over time to make things easier for people. I'm a middle child, a fixer- a peacemaker. The one who looks up to their older siblings, to grow up like them and tries to be a good role model for the younger one. Tries to toe the line of being good and doing right. I had an unusual last name as a kid; I had unusual curly hair and a flat chest by junior high standards. I learned how to make these things my own, use them to disarm people, if I acknowledged them- they weren't hurtful, or were they?

People ask how you are. They make observations- how you walk, talk, move and eat. If you do it well, they might think cancer is easy. Thing is- they only see you on the days you decide to go out prepared. They don't always see the "other" days that your family has to support your efforts.

When I had to go thru chemo the first time, I couldn't see myself wearing a hair prosthesis, the official medical term for a wig. I figured- if someone knew I was follicularly impaired I was being honest, I didn't know I could trust a wig to stay on my head. Having it fall off in front of a patient would be so embarrassing, plus how freaked out would they be? So I'm not wiggin' out this time either.

I know I've probably read somewhere about changing your outlook or presentation alters your own outlook and feelings. We'll go with that. I'm not a princess. I do like pink, but high heels, nail polish and dressing up are rare occasions. Give me jeans, a sweatshirt and some sneakers and I'm a happy girl.

These days it takes a little more to make me feel

presentable. The outfit takes time. The lack of breasts makes a difference in what you choose. No, I don't have to wear a bra, but I don't like to flaunt my lack of mammary tissue either. It's a layering-masking task. A tank or cami with a light sweater or shirt. Throw a scarf around the neck? Well, depends what I'm wearing up top. Got to cover the noggin now. A scarf? A do-rag? Hat? Hat with cute little flower on the side? You know people really go for those!

By the time I've gotten dressed, I feel like I'm about to go on stage. I can put on my super-M persona, drive to town and talk to almost anyone about my diagnosis, prognosis and treatment regimen. It's nice they notice I look good, but I don't feel it deep down. More than likely, if you see me out of the house, I'll tell you, "It's a good day" (physically) and you'll believe me. Whether I believe it is another story...

Over the next few months, a few new symptoms came up: strange red rash skin areas, skin sensitive to sunlight, hands and feet swelling or tingling, greyish skin on heels, difficulty with dexterity, weakness, visual changes, bloody nose. Courses of steroids were ordered. My weight crept up nearly fifteen pounds.

What kept me going? Knowing each round brought me closer to finishing treatment.

On 8-14-2011, my childhood friend wrote, "I think I would like to refer to you, from time to time, as the Irrepressible M. I read it in a book dedication and I think the shoe really fits! :)"

A few days after my fifth round of chemo, I felt horrible and had a hard time mentally functioning. When my temperature rose, we went to the emergency room at the order of the oncologist on call. The lab results showed I was neutropenic. My body was unable to fight an infection, so they admitted me for IV antibiotics. My lab work also showed my low energy: potassium was low, and Hemoglobin was near 8 (normal range is 12-15). I needed to have two units of blood transfused. I bounced back in a few days.

Even though I felt well enough to go home, I still felt the effects of the chemo regimen. I bruised easily. The medical staff wanted to wait longer to administer my last chemo, which worked out for the best in the end.

That happened the week of the big pink race in the city. Lots of people from my husband's work, my friends from work, family, and a couple of high school friends flew in to walk with me. We walked, and the next week I completed chemo.

A few weeks later, October 2011, I was back at work. My manager had called before my return to give me a heads-up. The company that had acquired our facility was reviewing the number of extended leave absences, questioning return or dismissal of those staff members. I had been out just over six months and was happy to be back. I was fortunate to have such a caring manager and coworkers. Except for wearing do-rags on my noggin, I felt pretty normal for the first time in months.

11

GET YOUR SHIT TOGETHER

Journal entry Valentine's Day 2012 (sitting in a coffee shop): *People coming and going. Normally I can't concentrate with so much going on around me. I say that because it's been months since I even opened a file for more than 5 minutes. Easier to write here and stay objective. I have to write this stuff down and deal with it before Thursday. Wrap my head around it and flush it out. Purge.*

I'm teary eyed and that shit needs to stop right now. At home I'd probably be bawling. Not a great thing to be sobbing in public...had my pre-op this morning...Happy Valentine's Day. In two days I get my bricks, I mean tissue expanders.

If someone told me 20 years ago I'd be having surgery to get breast implants, I'd have laughed. Ha, ha, ha. Back then I was going to college, newly married and we were lucky to make it paycheck to paycheck. I wasn't well endowed, but I had enough and it wasn't something that someone like me needed or wanted. Breast implants. Ha!

The thing is I'm not having augmentation. It's reconstruction. Starting from little more than piles of fat around the divots where my boobs used to be. Going back through the mastectomy scars, lifting up the pectoral and serratus muscles, placing an inflatable implant, drains and stitching it all shut. Over the next months I'll get "pumped up" then exchange surgery for the regular implants.

I feel conflicted. I can rationalize the surgery. It's not augmentation. It is reconstruction after breast cancer and mastectomy. In fact, federal law mandates insurance companies to pay for it, allowing me to restore to aid in my psychological healing, maybe even getting back to normal. I have a new normal, one that won't let me forget what happened, what I've gone through and what could possibly happen in the future.

Having this surgery is like starting all over again. I feel the same way I did last year when I got the second diagnosis. Ok it is not being vain, it is attempting to restore what was taken from me... I'm sure there are other types of cancer that can physically change your appearance. But breast cancer? It can take the boobs, the hair and the sense of well-being...The boobs are gone. The normal feeling, sensitivity and even the nipple are gone. The mounds can be replaced. Even nipple-like structures can be made. Tattoos can simulate the tissue pigmentation of the areola and nipple. But it will never be the same.

No one has actually come up to me and asked about my lack of breast tissue. I figure, either I don't get out much, people already know, people assume I don't have much or they really don't notice. I notice. I choose my clothes very carefully. Layers and dark colors are my camouflage. But vests and sweaters can be unbearable in Oklahoma. But I'm sure some will notice the growth and changes over the next few months...

I n February 2012, I started the breast reconstruction process. The plastic surgeon placed tissue expanders under my pectoral muscles. The expanders allow periodic filling with saline to grow pocket space for implants, breast prosthesis.

Journal entry: *There are days where you couldn't have written the strange events or coincidence. I wore my comfortable clothes to the hospital, grey Oklahoma hoodie, grey sweatpants and sneakers. On the highway exit ramp for the hospital and what song starts to play on the radio? The Rocky theme, "Flyin' high now" and we start to laugh. Before I disrobed for surgery, I threw my hands up to sky and my husband caught a picture of his Rocky.*

The surgery went well. I woke up in a room with my husband at my bedside. He later went to get the kids. Some nursing students tried to assist me to the bathroom to void. Then they stayed. They stood there. Waiting for me to go. I understand safety and all that. But hells bells- my bladder is shy and doesn't like an audience. I eke out a few drops. There. Happy?

My upper torso is wrapped in ace bandages. Drainage tubes poked out and little grenade shaped drains were pinned to my gown. So when I got queasy, I said, "Oh this is gonna suck," and puked. I fully woke up about bedtime. I rested, woke for the bathroom and would walk a little bit in the hall. I was doing pretty well & my doctor sent me home the next morning.

Since the expanders were put there to be "pumped up," I referred to them as "Hans and Franz." It was a small homage to the characters from the *Saturday Night Live* skit years ago.

If you think growing boobs the first time was awkward, doing it at 40 years old is even stranger. Let me tell you, they are not "free boobs." If you have a self-image issue, breast cancer is not the way to improve your bust—quite the opposite. My range of motion was limited. To get in the correct position for the saline fill, I lay on the exam table and had to lift one arm using the other to push at my elbow until the hand was above my head. Then I had to maintain that position for a few minutes as the breast was wiped with antiseptic and then pierced with a needle for the saline to be delivered into the tissue expander.

The plastic surgeon said I was doing rather well considering some augmentation patients would arrive to appointments using a wheelchair from the lobby, whereas, he noted, I walked in on my own two feet. In hindsight, I realize this was meant to be a compliment, albeit a back-assward one. How in the hell should I have acted given all I'd endured already? To me, you just can't compare reconstruction to augmentation—different patients with different issues entirely.

My right side developed red areas from pressure and thinning skin. The expansion process was put on hold. It looked and felt like I had turtle shells on my chest. The tissue expanders were hard, and each expansion caused upper back pain as the muscles tried to accommodate more volume underneath their surface.

Journal entry summer 2012: *Incisions healed well. Stripping drains TID (three times daily), little monkeys pinching my pits. Range of motion limited. Shiny skin after fills but can't feel it. Complicated year. Antibiotics for URI (upper respiratory infection) from PCP in January. Again for*

left arm cellulitis related to flu shot. Again post-op. Again for
unusual fever 3/1 from PCP. Fill 4/4 then overnight fever, see
PCP with labs, urine, chest x-ray, doxycycline prescription.
Cough & choke, fever breaks with sweating thru 2 pair
pajamas then shaking chills start. ER wait and wait, admit
over 90 minutes with [heart rate] 162 at triage. Chest x-ray,
CT- fluid behind expander, possible pneumonia. Red areas
develop, more antibiotics, possible pressure area. No further
fills.

In August 2012, I had the exchange surgery. Goodbye to "Hans and Franz," hello to the new girls, Frieda and Helga. The clear adhesive bandage applied after surgery overlapped at the center and lifted off my top layer of skin. That nickel-sized superficial skin injury took weeks to heal. With the healing process and the new implants, the red shiny areas had disappeared, making me think they had been pressure issues all along. The implants were not hard like the expanders, but there was a lack of cleavage. Instead of distinctive Frieda and Helga with a valley of cleavage between them, it was more like Frelga. I had a tube-like uniboob with just a slight divot in the middle. It was less than satisfactory results. When I questioned whether it could be fixed, my plastic surgeon replied that there was no guarantee it would work; in fact, it might be worse.

His response gave me the impression that what I had was as good as it was going to get. So I went home to start my next chapter of life with Frelga. After all, I was happily married and my husband was the only one who would see me undressed, and he was thankful I was alive.

Over time, the discomfort of the uniboob named Frelga became more disruptive. Wide sweeping arm movements made my whole chest twitch and shift. I could not tolerate hand weights or any upper-body, weight-bearing exercises. The process of wiping a table, sweeping, vacuuming, lifting items, or reaching for objects always felt awkward for me. And the implants become harder.

In 2013, my oncologist started me on a medication named Femara to block any estrogen sources in my body. The plan was to be on it for five years. I did have the hysterectomy, but your body can make hormones that mimic estrogen. There are also products you ingest or use that can be like estrogen to your body, so the medication blocks them from fueling a new cancer. It sounded good enough. Then I noticed more fatigue, foot and hand pains, joint pains, and increased irritability. I experienced weird chest pains, as well as left arm and neck pain, but it was blocking cancer, right?

For more than two and a half years, I put up with Frelga. We had changed insurance companies and I requested a consult with the plastic surgeon that my general surgeon had originally recommended (my previous insurance didn't cover him). Finally able to meet this plastic surgeon, I was impressed with just one visit. What I was experiencing was called capsular contracture and symmastia. *It was a real medical problem!* Capsular contraction was scar tissue formation that squeezed and caused shape change to the implants. Symmastia was muscle damage when too large of an implant is used in the pocket, tearing the muscle from the sternum, or the muscle is cut too much and later rips. This doctor told me he'd seen about twenty cases in his thirty years of practice. It was not an issue in his practice, because it just didn't happen with his patients. It might not be an easy fix, but we could make my chest look and feel better.

I discussed the surgery with my oncologist. I certainly trusted her after so many years together. I also discussed my frustration with the Femara. We agreed to a drug holiday. After stopping the medication, my symptoms improved. We went on a road trip to a great amusement park where I rode nearly every roller coaster and then went to see family. It was summertime and I felt good.

The thought of starting over again with tissue expanders wasn't exciting, but the possibility of ending the twitch, shift, and discomfort was encouraging.

Frelga exited my chest in July 2015. The muscles were repaired and tacked down, while the pocket was enlarged and new tissue expanders were placed.

In the past, I have had weird surgical recovery issues, like not being able to urinate or not being able to wake up enough to walk. That's kind of a big deal before you go home.

After this surgery, the recovery nurse kept asking, "Are you ready to go home?"

Even in my drug-induced stupor, I was getting irritated and responded, "You know, I don't know, usually I'm much more decisive!" At that point, my husband advised her to call the doctor about my post-op issues.

The medical staff transferred me to a room to stay overnight until my plumbing worked again. My next nurse on the floor joked way too much. I motioned to my husband that I wanted to stab myself in the eye with a pen, just so someone else would have to come in the room. I admit, that wasn't my greatest idea and I certainly didn't do it. The pain medication made my groin and lower back itch like crazy! Also, I saw flies where I knew there weren't any. My husband dared to joke about the phantom flies that night, but I'd had enough and it wasn't funny to me. It's the only time I've ever said f--- you to him. Later, I apologized. It may have been the flies, the meds, and the pain, or wearing my hair in braids while channeling my inner Ronda Rousey or all of the above, but it was not one of my proudest moments. But I'll own it, because shit happens.

Recovery at home was so much different. I had no drains

and hardly any pain. I did have to wear a special thong-like bra with a roll of gauze between the breasts to keep the repaired cleavage from lifting. Another not-so-sexy moment in my life. And then I had some shingles pop up.

But what a difference in sensation. No turtle shells—these expanders were more like tough automotive sponges, durable with a little give. I dubbed them "Thing 1" and "Thing 2."

Then it was time to see the oncologist. I had to see a different doctor, since mine was away on leave. This doctor was nice but spoke plainly. She insisted I needed to be on something to block estrogen. Let's try a different hormone blocker, rather than risk a recurrence of cancer. I started Aromasin and hoped to tolerate it better.

I went back to work in the beginning of September 2015. Every few weeks, I'd have an appointment to add volume to the expanders, allowing my pectorals to stretch and accommodate the change. It was going really well, and by Christmas, I had the biggest bosom in my life.

In February 2016, we noticed a volume loss on the right side, which would require replacing the volume for symmetry before going to exchange surgery.

We finally scheduled the exchange surgery for June 2016. It was at a different hospital than the last time. I had to use special antibacterial surgical prep wipes at home, after showering before bed the night before surgery. When I woke up in the morning, I was to use the wipes again. We had an afternoon surgery time, and with no eating before surgery, my husband feared for the staff as I tend to get hangry.

I checked in for the surgery and paid my insurance deductible. The staff led me to pre-op and told me to wipe down yet again. So there I was, naked behind a curtain and balancing on my shoes to wipe myself down, while not touching anything or falling, and waiting for the moisture to air dry before donning my surgery gown and bonnet. After that process, the anesthesia team dropped by. They moved my backpack from the chair where I'd placed it and set it on the floor so they could sit. They didn't ask me.

SET MY BAG ON THE FLOOR?! IN A HOSPITAL?!

My husband picked up the backpack and set it elsewhere, hoping I would allow the five-second rule, but that rule doesn't apply in a hospital setting. Ever. I really did need anesthesia, so I kept my trap shut.

Then a nurse stopped by to start my IV.

"Well, with a history of bilateral mastectomy, we'll have to use a foot," she said.

"Yeah, we're not doing that," I replied.

My husband told me later that he heard my tone and clicked off checking his work emails to watch how it would play out.

The nurse started my IV in my left arm on the first try—best one I've ever had. That must have been some pressure, but it was my right as a patient to refuse. I knew my body, and I had no history of lymph node removal on my left side and no lymphedema issues. But I did have issues with foot pain. My feet were always cold, so good luck getting a vein down there. I didn't need complications in my feet.

I don't recall much after surgery. My husband said we closed the bar down, last patient to leave that day around dinner time. I had some vomiting into a puke-tube baggie before wheeling out to the truck and sleeping on the ride home. My husband made me some cream of wheat, and I nibbled on popsicles only to power-puke a short time later. The anesthesia finally wore off, so I was wide awake at 10 p.m.

My surgeon saw me the next day, and my binder and dressing were removed. There was swelling on the left and the right was sliding to the side, kind of wonky and puckered. And I had no drains. The doctor told me to use the thong bra, shower, and pat dry. I could transition to a special underwire sports bra to aid in proper placement of the implants. I was skeptical since I'd not been able to wear an underwire for years because of discomfort after my lumpectomy in 2003. This bra was different though, with the well-padded underwire on the outside of the cups and positioned around the breasts. There was also a special pressure strap applied higher on the chest, above the breast implants, to keep them low in the pocket.

At three days post-op, both of my kids had plans to leave the house.

I said, "Go ahead."

They both paused, looked at each other, some unstated conversation happening between them. They fessed up that Dad had told them not to leave me alone. At 44 years old, I had to have a baby sitter?

So I texted him: *Is there any way you would allow me to stay home alone without a sitter for a few hours this afternoon? She has to work and he was going to hang out with friends. If no then I will sit at the coffee shop with her until he is done hanging out and can come get me. I promise not to lift anything but a cup or a utensil to my mouth- or not if you don't want me to. I will not go outside or drive my Jeep and will not answer the door or pay any attention at all to the dogs. Hershey can drop a ripe old deuce and it will wait for the kids if that's what it takes... I have not taken any pain or mind altering meds since yesterday afternoon. Please? Pretty please?!? Actually that's a lie, no pain meds since Wednesday.*

He replied, "Only this once."

He then added, "I laughed out loud, so did everyone else-that was top 10 material." He shared my text request with all the guys in the office. They probably think, poor guy—she's a nut!

Recovery went well over the next few weeks, and I went back to work.

At that time, Hershey was our oldest dog. She was a chocolate lab, with a great temperament, and followed directions very well until she became hard of hearing. You could tell she was losing her vision too, as her eyes became more cloudy or she missed treats thrown in her direction. She'd had ligament surgery on both back legs, and she'd survived a life-threatening spider or snake bite. She'd also survived heartworms and had constant ear infections. Over the years, she became slower and stiffer. Around that time, she had a hard time getting up. She would lift her front but struggle with her back end. She would tense up, trying to lift herself, and sometimes dribble urine or lose some poop out her back end. She was still happy, ate well, and would bark if she needed out. The barking increased, as did the poop episodes.

At the end of August 2016, I had what was supposed to be a simple eye procedure. My recovery took a little longer than expected. On a Thursday afternoon, I let Hershey and the other two dogs out.

Hershey lay down near the shed. She couldn't hear or see me calling her. Her back end had gotten wedged under the bottom of the shed. I started to nudge her out with my toes. I don't know if she didn't hear me, see me, or sense me, but she whipped her head around fast. I stepped back. There was no growl or snap, but that moment made me realize that it was time.

If she hurt someone because she couldn't hear or see them coming, or if she was hurting and someone tried to lift her, could I live with that?

I got her back end up, and she ambled to the house. The

next day, she could not stand on her own at all. The day after that, we said goodbye at her final veterinarian appointment. We had her cremated and she rests next the fireplace, her favorite spot, to this day.

Putting down a dog can make you examine your own quality of life. She'd had so many challenges and survived things that other owners would have used as reasons to put her down, rather than pay for treatments. That dang dog reminded me so much of myself. We'd both endured more than the usual share of health issues.

There have been some really strange things in my medical history. In my teenage years, I had chemical abrasions on my corneas due to contact lenses twice. Shortly after we married, I was treated for strange joint pain and discoloration, twice, which was diagnosed as Lyme disease. A rheumatologist diagnosed me with Sjogren's Syndrome, an autoimmune disorder associated with joint pain, dry eyes and mouth. Over the years, I'd had issues with map-dot fingerprinting dystrophy erosions which led to my eye surgery that August. Then breast cancer twice and the two reconstruction surgeries.

I'd addressed my own quality-of-life issues over the last few years. Getting rid of Frelga was a start. The major surgery, expansion, and exchange took patience and considerable time to avoid complications. The medication holiday and change also alleviated some of my unusual aches and pains. My quality had improved considerably.

Almost four months post-op, I requested an appointment. The right-side implant seemed higher and tighter. The doctor put me on a few medications to soften the tissue and hopefully prevent capsular contracture. We discussed revision surgery.

Over the next few months, there was only slight improvement of the implant, but I had developed numbness, pain, and tingling down my right arm to my hand and fingers. My upper back and neck were always tight. I felt the need to stretch, to adjust my posture and back all the time. My upper spine would pop and give me a short reprieve.

The doctor suggested more medication and I tried it. In the few days of tapering up the dose, I could not tolerate it. There was no way I could live or work in a "buzzed" state. You know the feeling when you've had a few drinks; the world seems to slow down, sounds are slightly muffled, and you are a bit more careful how you walk. That might be enjoyable on a night out, but not for a lifetime, or even months.

It was seven months since surgery for the new implants. In hindsight, I realized they had not been named. A friend suggested "Thelma and Louise" or "Laverne and Shirley." Although both were great suggestions, neither one seemed to fit. My body just didn't want them. Maybe that's why no names ever seemed to "fit." I talked with my husband and kids. I'd made a decision and was done with reconstruction.

My surgery to remove the implants and hopefully alleviate my discomfort issues was scheduled. I told my siblings and coworkers. They all encouraged me to do whatever I had to in order to be comfortable again. They had witnessed the process, but were not aware of all the problems that led to my decision.

Even though I looked normal in clothes, the implants did not feel or move like natural breasts. Natural breasts hang a bit as you age and they can be manipulated so you can wash or check the underside. The left one could be shifted manually a little, but the right was harder and tight. I could not see my feet without bending at the waist. The only way to explain the sensation of my chest with implants was to imagine a set of cold grapefruit duct taped to your chest. I have never been a fan of grapefruit.

Even though cancer had taken my breasts, I had tried for a long time to look normal for my family, friends, and society in general. It didn't work the first time due to the compromised muscles, and my body surely didn't like the implants the second time. Post-op recovery after implant removal was the best yet. They had used different medications to manage my anesthesia, nausea, and pain. The duct-taped grapefruit sensation was gone. Within a few days, I knew the upper back problem was resolved. I could breathe easier. Sleeping was more comfortable. It was a new sort of freedom for me.

12

SHITHEADS

M y first word of advice if you have a loved one or friend going through possible cancer diagnosis or during their treatment: don't be a shithead. Don't give some false hope. Don't deny the possibility they might have cancer. Don't downplay or minimize the situation because of your discomfort, or they may want to come back and throttle you.

Support them. Allow them the choice to discuss their experience if they want to do that. Ask about upcoming appointments, whether someone is going with them. Encourage them to write down questions to ask the doctor for their peace of mind. A second set of ears is helpful to recall details and ask pertinent questions.

Use caution in your choice of words and actions. They can make jokes about their cancer and looks. You should not. For example, I can say my aspirations to be a stripper or pole dancer are over, obviously, without a set of breasts to be oogled. That statement from anyone else—they sound like an ass. The euphemisms for breasts might be funny to some, yet offensive to others. Some people don't mind pink-ribbon

76

themed gifts, while others don't want a daily reminder of their stalker and potential killer. Some people will walk or race for the pink ribbon, while others want to fly under the radar—even from family, friends, and work.

I've had a few shithead encounters, people who made me feel worse for no good reason. Maybe they're oblivious to the wording of the questions or comments and the effect it has on a patient or their family. I'm going to play devil's advocate believing that, rather than think the intent was malicious.

On the day of my MUGA in January 2004, I was at a facility for a nursing school clinical day. I was dressed as a student nurse. At the time of my appointment, I arrived at the patient waiting area and signed in with the reception clerk. A nurse took me back to a room, asked the usual admitting questions, and started an IV. I was taken to radiology with my orders in hand. I rested under a special x-ray machine for a little while and then it was done. My IV was taken out, and I was dismissed.

After the MUGA, I went back to the outpatient reception to schedule my bone scan. The clerk stated there were no orders for that test, so she couldn't schedule it.

Yes, there were orders. I had seen them that morning on the same sheet that I had handed over to the radiology technician for the MUGA. So I went back to radiology and asked for a copy of the orders. The tech graciously paused for my request, copied the orders, and highlighted the additional test to be scheduled in yellow.

When I went back to the clerk with that paper, she said "That wasn't on there this morning."

Basically, she accused me of writing my own orders! First, no one would choose to have a bone scan just for the fun of it. Second, writing a doctor's orders for testing without a physician's direction to do so could get you in serious trouble and possibly end a career before it even began.

I tried to explain that the original paper was with the radiology technician. She told me she couldn't schedule it, that I had to go to scheduling in the business office. First, she had only told me there were no orders. Then when confronted with a lapse in scheduling, she said the order wasn't on the sheet previously. Now she was piling on the difficulty and making me go elsewhere. I'd like to think she was just having a bad day, rather than being chronically nasty. I made my way to the business office cubicles, where a nice lady named Debbie assisted me and apologized for the clerk's accusation.

Shithead encounters can be unintentional and from unlikely sources.

An awkward encounter happened at church. Before the service, some people visit just outside the sanctuary before going in to sit. One elderly member, whom I didn't know, stopped me to talk. With a do-rag on my head, I was the obvious cancer patient in our church and on the prayer list because of the cancer treatment. This person asked how I was doing and *did they get it all?*

"Excuse me?"

I did not know this person, had never met them, and they were inquiring about my prognosis?! At that moment, I felt they were really asking: *So, are you a lost cause? Or do we keep ya on the prayer list?* That's probably not what this person intended, but that was my perception.

After the service, I told my husband about the exchange. He listened and got quiet for a few minutes. He then told me we were done with church for a while. People didn't need to be asking about my personal business and I shouldn't be around all those germs. He wanted to protect me from the words and the world. He knows I am a person who will stew on a situation, then possibly blow up on it, so he was also protecting others from my wrath.

When you have cancer, some people just don't know what to say. They tell you stories about their friend's mother's sister who had cancer and is now fine. They don't mention what treatment was used or how old the person was at the time.

Comparing cancer stories is like comparing fruits to vegetables. They may have common colors, they come from the same department in the store, and you eat them, but they vary in fiber and vitamin content. Some people start a story because it is cancer related, because they know someone who had it. They recall some vague treatment of surgery, chemo, radiation, or natural healing which the patient endured, and then they died. That is not helpful. Less is more. Hold the horror stories when you're not one who is dealing with cancer.

In June 2004, I attended a local cancer walk with my nursing school instructors and classmates. By that time, I was in radiation treatment, still bald and wearing a do-rag. I wore a t-shirt I'd been given at radiation that week that exclaimed on the back, "HAD IT. FOUGHT IT. SURVIVED IT." Throughout the evening, there were many questions and introductions—I was exhausted. At one point, they encouraged "survivors" to come forward for special recognition of the cancer type and how longer they'd been in remission. I felt very much alone being much younger than most and not knowing any of them.

A group of older women inquired, "What kind of cancer did you have?" Having answered that same question numerous times already in a single day, I felt cornered, defensive really, and gave them a shithead answer.

"Boobie."

They didn't ask anything else and slinked away. Not my finest moment.

Years later, when I was going to have the mastectomy, I

encountered a few more shitheads. There I was, about to have my breasts amputated, and some people thought they were helping me see the glass as half full by saying, "Well, you get to have some free boobs."

They're not free. I paid. Insurance paid.

"Yours will be perkier than mine!"

Seriously? Implied jealousy on reconstruction after mastectomy for breast cancer? Well, maybe they can be jealous that reconstruction implants will be perky—like even after I'm dead, they'd still be perky.

"Are you gonna get some big ones?"

That must be the one upside to breast cancer that people assume. Oh my. Big fake boobs fix nothing and complicate everything. If I heard that line one more time, I was seriously going to lose my shit!

Humor is often a way to deflect pain. Breasts and cancer are uncomfortable topics—I get that. But that was *their* humor about *my* pain. And it wasn't funny at all. Think about it: would anyone make those kinds of statements about any other cancer surgery?

In 2011, the facility I worked for was acquired by another hospital system. We had to reapply for the benefits we already had for the transition to new insurance policies. My benefit papers were completed and submitted on time, while I was still on medical leave for treatment.

Two months after the sale was finalized and I'd been back at work for a month, I was notified through the mail by the insurance carrier that I was ineligible for coverage. Turns out, having a history of cancer works against you when you want death and disability insurance. But the happy, little bean-counting wench on the end of the phone told me I could reapply... in five years.

I asked her if she knew the statistics about breast cancer.

She said, "1 in 8 women will be affected in their lifetime."

I replied, "That's right. Since I've had it twice, consider it once for me and once for you, Bitch! I hope you NEVER have to walk in MY SHOES!"

Understand just a few things here—I was not a new employee since my company had been acquired by another. Applying for benefits was a formality, since I'd already had accidental death and disability coverage in place. Since the time of the official acquisition, money for benefits had been deducted from my payroll check, with two months of premium already paid. When I shared my issue with Human Resources, they were able to make the insurance company understand the situation a bit clearer. My benefits were confirmed.

I'd like to pause a moment and make a point. It's been over seven years of premium paid into the plan. I was just a number on a file, a statistic, rejected due to a negative response that didn't fit in the flow diagram and denied without regard to my personal situation. I had to argue and fight to pay that money. Who's the benefactor now? *You're welcome!*

Moral of the story: think before you speak or act. Don't be a shithead to someone with cancer.

13

TOUGH SHIT

"How are yoooouuuuu?" The question was unusually long and drawn out to convey compassion or concern by the asker. Their eyes darted to the chest area at some point during the encounter. Comments were made about my sassy hair growing back and how young it made me look.

"You look soooo goooooooddd." Again, drawn out to convey concern and compassion. While I appreciate the compliment, have I not looked goooooooddd every other day? I really do work on my appearance, but to think one day was that much better than the rest made me wonder if I got dressed in the dark sometimes.

"You're so brave." No, I'm really not brave at all.

"You're so strong." No, I'd say I'm tough and developed a thicker skin out of necessity.

"I don't think I could do it." I didn't have a choice.

I couldn't just throw up my hands and say, "I'm done—cancer has won." Not when you have two children, a husband, and others who count on you.

"How do you do it?" Juggling treatment, home, and school

wasn't easy with my first diagnosis, but I only missed one day back then. My five-year plan was to finish LPN school, earn a Bachelor of Science in Nursing, and become a registered nurse. Done, done, and done.

There is no doubt in my mind that the second time was harder. I was older, wiser in some ways, and it was more of a physical challenge with two major surgeries. This book became my new five-year plan. (Admittedly, I'm a little late on that, but remember I was creatively constipated!)

Have you ever heard that a person is never given more than what they can handle? We don't have to agrcc as to whether that statement is true, only that you may have heard it.

Think of the times when your plate is so full—those times when you think you can't possibly pile on anything else, because gravy is starting to dribble off on one side, while your biscuit is barely balanced on the other. And yet, you need to hold onto that fork. When you make a happy plate and the table is cleared, there is supposed to be some kind of fabulous dessert!

I'll tell you what I've told my friends and some of my own patients. You deal with one thing at a time. I actually have to stop and remind myself at times. When I have a bunch to do, a list helps me know what I've yet to do and what I have accomplished. You start with one manageable task. Feel good when you complete it and set another goal. Sounds easy, right?

Not so long ago, a patient confided that since a major event and surgery in her life, she was depressed. She had no energy to do things, no joy, and lived in fear. In nursing school, they don't teach you what to say to a person going through this, but I'll tell you what I said and it seemed to help. I shared my own personal illness history. I'd had my first bout with cancer, went through surgeries, chemo, and radiation. Every six months for seven years, I'd had to face the machines and the oncologist's office to get my a-okay for another six months. I advised her to speak with her doctor about the depression and we called to make an appointment. We also spoke about how far she'd come since her event and surgery.

"Small victories are still victories. Celebrate them and you." I encouraged her to wake up and get ready for the day. Plan and cook a favorite recipe to share with a loved one. Make an appointment to do something and keep it. Get the prescription for an antidepressant and fill it. One task at a time.

After my second diagnosis, I happened to run into that same patient. We talked and celebrated how far she had come and how encouraged we were by each other.

Being a nurse and a patient, having to wear both pairs of shoes—sometimes on the same day—I know what I aspire to do for people who step into the door of my facility, not just my patients. Just like anywhere else, healthcare worker personalities run the complete spectrum. Just like with patients, healthcare workers have lives outside of work, as well as families and worries of their own. There are dedicated, hardworking, and emotionally involved employees on one end, while over yonder are others who openly discuss anything but the patient in front of their patients. You've known the type: rules are rules, you are just a number on a file, and they're just there for their paycheck every two weeks.

In the LPN program, there were required educational training videos and movies to better understand healthcare experiences. A few films I'd highly recommend to anyone in healthcare: *The Doctor*, *The Bucket List*, and *The Fault in Our Stars*. Until you've had your own near-death experience, you can't comprehend the patient's perception of their diagnosis and appreciate their personal situation.

Sometimes people, even healthcare workers, forget that with illness there is anxiety, pain, and an altered outlook; sometimes a person is changed forever. Once there has been a major illness, for that person, the mind goes back to *what if it's happening again?* Patients might call or show up frequently or early for appointments. Patients don't know or understand everything they are dealing with, how a facility operates, or the medications sent home with them. Everyone should agree that there are no stupid questions. For their sake, if you say you'll call back, follow up and do it. Otherwise, you may be the recipient of unkind words related to their anxiety. Have patience with your patients.

There have been a number of times over the years when people have reached out to me for information when they had a breast concern or recent diagnosis. There were emails, phone calls, and meetings to discuss their situations. There is no doubt that each of them had family and friends to call upon in their time of need, but no one gets it quite like someone who "gets it."

This was an email (2-24-2013) to a friend's friend about breast surgery:

I know we talked briefly about breast reconstruction concerns. For someone who has a family history, have they personally been BRCA tested? That is the genetic test to see if in fact they are a carrier. It should be done prior to considering all the surgery. If they are not a carrier, but have a strong family history and have been advised to have prophylactic bilateral mastectomy, will insurance cover the surgery and have there been any second or third opinions?

Reconstruction can occur for some people at the time of

mastectomy (immediate) but there will be two surgeons- one for the mastectomy and the other for reconstruction, and they will have to coordinate the procedures.

Mastectomy is removal of all the breast tissue, the top layer of the pectoral may also be removed to ensure all breast tissue is gone. The nipple and areola complex may also be taken- depends on the doctor and patient. They consider future risk basically.

Reconstruction options include transplanting your own muscle tissue (from either the tummy, back or buttocks) or implants placed under the pectoral muscles. If there haven't been previous implants, tissue expanders may be used to expand a pocket to allow implants when the desired size is reached. Implants are more common from what I've read and simpler. Harvesting and moving the muscles takes long surgery and it isn't done everywhere around the country. Anywhere muscle is harvested from there will be scars, and possibility of hernia or loss of range of motion.

Some people do choose not to have reconstruction also.

It is a lengthy process. Recovery from the surgeries takes anywhere from 6 weeks to much longer if there are any complications.

Throughout the process it is important to really like the doctor, because you'll be seeing them a lot. Ask to see some of their work. It should be something they offer to educate the patient on what to expect for the process and outcome.

Just read this to my hubby and he couldn't think of anything to add. He was a great source of support as you know and a person going through recon will need help with transport to appointments, help with recovery at home, chores, etc...

Best wishes to the reader of this email as you forward it...

My doctor's office called to ask if I would consider talking to a lady who was recently diagnosed with her second breast cancer. They thought I might be able to lend some insight about going through another diagnosis, mastectomy, and reconstruction. I encouraged them to share my contact information and leave it up to her to go from there. We talked by phone, then I sent the following email on 3-1-2015:

There are so many things I could tell you based on what I went through, but each person's experience is a bit different. The following tips are just about mastectomy (chemo came later). Keep in mind- you are stronger than you realize, people are available to help you and they want to, so take them up on it!

Prior to surgery: Keep appointments for the doctor, consults, tests and pre-op check-in. You may be given literature or handouts- a folder is good to keep it all together and have your questions written down too. Gather some loose fitting tops (button up or zip up are great) and elastic waist bottoms, slip on shoes. These things go on easily without too much overhead arm movement or tugging. Not having to bend over to tie shoes or fit them over your heel is helpful. When people ask what they can do or "call me if I can help," give them a task. As simple as: pray for me, a meal would be great, e-mail me, needing a ride, etc. They care, yet don't want to intrude. Sometimes it is hard to ask for help, so when it is offered- take them up on it...

There are websites where you can set up a private central messaging place for you or your family to manage. Rather than taking calls, repeating details- you can privately post to people that have internet access through a page and password you set up. It can be as private as you want it to be.

I was of the mindset- if I know all possibilities, even worst case, then anything else is better. But how much you want to know is entirely up to you. The internet is bound to pull up tons of pages on breast cancer, but not all of it is entirely reliable based on the source... There are many people with different experiences and they ARE NOT doctors. ALWAYS RELY ON YOUR OWN DOCTOR FOR MEDICAL ADVICE OR CONTACT THEM ABOUT YOUR CONCERNS.

Ask what is needed to bring to the hospital and pack it in a bag (family can hold it for you). Place things that you are allowed to use post-op within reach at waist level (kitchen and bathroom items). There will be a few limitations for a few days on weight and manipulation of some things, a little longer on others like running the vacuum...

Do things you enjoy, treat yourself to a fun day every now and then, use a journal to jot down your thoughts and write down concerns to ask about. After surgery: REST, do what your doctor advises and take your medications as directed when needed. You'll be taught how to care for your drains and dressing. Follow up appointments will be scheduled. They'll tell you what to report to the doctor and pain medications may be prescribed for home. Have a notepad near your medications and dressing care area. Writing down the amount of drain fluid and when you took medications is important. That way you can easily recall the details when needed. Until you are cleared to shower, you will have to sponge bathe. Someone who can assist with this is great, or you can use baby wipes/personal cleansing cloths. Since your reach is limited- the hair will have to be done by someone too, but only for a few days.

For all the people I could relate to—those who have been there or close to it—I can also share a view into the "what if this doesn't go well" mindset. My family and friends were always supportive, and I can recall only one discussion we had of the possibility of treatment failure. It was with the person who had seen me at my best and worst over the years, my husband.

He had taken off work to go to a regularly scheduled test with me.

Journal entry 3-17-2015: *...had a really honest conversation last week...We went to lunch...He told me- if I die before him he'd be at a loss on how to get thru the funeral, etc. Said he'd have to handle it with humor to cope. I suggested it too. We had a good laugh at saying he's not good talking to crowds so count off by 2s and half of you are outta here. At first I was shocked he's thought about it, but how can he not? My husband and my kids have seen all the rough stuff. Some family and friends know some of the details. Even other people with breast cancer have different perspectives because their treatment varied from mine. When faced with a challenge, you muddle through as best you can with whatever help you can get at the time, and hope for the best.*

My friend confided to me that she didn't understand how we coped at the time. She was frustrated that our family didn't come to stay during my surgeries. For half a second, I was shocked. It never occurred to me to ask family to come stay with us at the time, nor did I expect it. Hubby and I had raised the kids away from family for over a decade and understood it was hard for others to travel to us or leave their work and obligations. I was glad I had family and friends who reached out to support us. The captains of my long-distance support team were my mom and dad. They called us. Every day.

I'm tougher than I used to be—not brave or strong, which imply heroism to me. Not everyone diagnosed with cancer beats it, and it's not that they didn't try hard enough. To get through treatment requires perseverance against the odds, and one day at a time with a little help from family and friends.

"Coarse Adjustment"
(summer 2016 free verse poem)
How do you feel about sand in your toes?
Life is like that sand.
The cold rough stuff and the warm smooth stuff
shape and define a broken bottle
into a work of art over time.

14

MY GIVE A SHIT GOT BUSTED

People can agree that their relationships and their perception of the world changes with age. Cancer can do that for you too, real quick. It's not necessarily a process of maturing, but less tolerance for bullshit really.

So there you are, telling someone you have cancer. They most likely respond in one of three ways: supportive acceptance, shock and later avoidance, or the awkward divas. The best ones will just hug you, cry with you, bring you food, and check in on the family. The ones who just can't believe it, say you're their friend and they care so much, but that isn't always true. Some can't deal with it and pretty much fall off the edge of the Earth. Awkward divas want to get all up in your business and make it about them and what a good person they are—thank God I didn't have any of those.

The ones who fall of the edge? They really weren't a friend to begin with, if you think about it. Maybe at their own convenience they were, yes. They are so busy with work, family, kids, sports, volunteering, church, or carpooling, but they can't associate with their cancer-ridden friend. Probably because it hits too close to home. They want to float away, holding fast to their balloons of invincibility no matter what —even at the cost of what you thought was friendship. It wasn't. Let it go, you're better off without them.

One time, a "friend" said she'd come over to visit before I had surgery. Her family did. She didn't. She had to go shop with her committee that weekend for a work-related event.

A month later, after no calls and no visits, we met up at our community's cancer relay event. It was awkward just standing there and talking couple to couple.

A former patient's spouse walked by and pulled me aside to talk about their loved one. It was only a few minutes, but by then, my "friend" had left. My husband told me after her husband left that my pulling away to talk to someone else was rude. I explained that what happened was private and worked related. I thought maybe I should apologize to my "friend."

Initially, she acted like she didn't see me walk up to her group's booth. She admitted she'd heard I had surgery and asked, "*Did they get it all?*" Yep, she really asked that question after a double mastectomy. We chatted for a bit as I started to stew on that one question. Then we parted and she said to keep them informed, because (wait for it!) "*We care.*"

Oblivious, totally oblivious. That should be my priority, right? Contacting people to tell them all about my deficit of chest and soon to be exiting uterus too, right? Not focusing on getting well, caring for my family, or praying I'll make it through treatment.

Would you hang on to a friend like that, or let her go?

For years, I was rah-rah, pink everything—we'd walk to raise loads of money to help the cause. Over time, my view changed. Don't get me wrong, I still want to help people, but I'd rather do it on a personal basis.

Journal entry 3-27-2014: *...I'm not the same person I was...* *I'd been thinking about how much I'd lost. I'm glad to be alive but how much there has been to go through as well. I get pissed at little things like people asking- "Wanna buy a pink ribbon to support awareness?" NO! I'm aware. Tired of diseases being bastardized and people making money off of other's misery. That disgusts me. Funny-I have a pink Papermate "WRITE FOR HOPE" pen in my hand right now. It was given to me by someone who meant well and was just trying to be supportive. See that's the thing- people are guilted into getting these products or services they think are going to benefit research or people with the disease- but if you look very close at the labels- it's a flat dollar amount they donate- so if you buy 1 or 29 of something- it does NOT matter. Marketing assholes. So I have anger. I also try not to talk about my feelings or pain or thoughts too much. Not that I think people don't care, but I don't want pity or to make them feel bad. I just need to vent. So I debated going to a group for support. Thought about seeing a doctor, but I don't want to have a label of whatever diagnosis they think I have. When I went to Ohio I saw A's mom for the first time in years. She looked as though she would cry. BIG hug. I have that effect on people. Hadn't seen J since 2010 in Oklahoma. We had some talks: me, her and M. I have lost a lot. My body will never be the same. There is no good reason for all of this other than I had breasts. I think I've beat myself up enough on so many topics. Did I not exercise enough? Did I not eat well enough? Was it the tanning bed? Was it working in radio? Because another friend had it too. Was it some unknown gene? Was it to do with or not enough breastfeeding? Was it because of DES? And there's the whole concept of why a second time. Wonder if I was truly stage III first time and maybe that's why- more likely to occur again- but different. Through all of the treatment, surgery and all, I* *think I handled it all well. Maybe too well. I hate to cry. It makes it hard to breathe. But to talk to anyone I feel like I need to hold back. They don't know how it feels to lose yourself. And for a lot of the day I can go without thinking about it. But change my clothes, bathe, etc. the ugly facts rear their head. There's no escape. So how do you deal with all these feelings, thoughts?*

If you look at the big events held in communities all over the country to raise funds, they advocate "AWARENESS" campaigns. Various companies donate products or locations to the event for the cause. Guess what? It's also a tax write-off for them, not just generosity to the survivors. If you participate, you paid a charge to get your "free" t-shirt. Been there, done that, and had way too many t-shirts.

At one point, I was so frustrated and refused to be a walking billboard anymore by wearing the t-shirts. I got rid of all of them, except the very first that read, "HAD IT. FOUGHT IT. SURVIVED IT." I ordered my own special t-shirt. It is dark grey with a hot pink stenciled font reading "Been there, done that, got the t-shirt."

The amount of money spent on logoed supplies, mailings, advertising, and general stuff is overwhelming. The budget going to research, patient care, and assistance versus payroll boggles the mind. If you aren't convinced yet, watch *Pink Ribbons Inc.*

Don't forget October is breast cancer awareness month. Stores and websites are splattered with pink-ribboned products. Clerks pester customers for donations at the register because it's a corporate directive. Companies use the pink ribbon as marketing strategy on all sorts of products (pepper spray, guns, eggs, coffee cups, pens, socks, clothes) so you think you're helping, but how much did it really help anyone outside of that particular company? Read the fine print. Only a portion of the proceeds, capped at a certain dollar amount, will be given to the yada-yada-yada fund. Again, it's a donation and tax write-off. They "give" to pimp the pink ribbon while boosting sales and making money off other people's misery.

Have people become numb to the pink ribbon?

Think of all the catchy slogans used regarding breast cancer. At one time, I thought they were cute too or I just tried to ignore them. Then it hit too close to home, at my own workplace, and I had to respond to that insult through official channels.

Memo e-mailed to Human Resources 9-28-2015:

Statistics show breast cancer affects 1 in 8 women in her lifetime. Mammograms are an important screening tool, so I understand the campaign to encourage and remind women of early detection, but question the t-shirt slogan chosen and approved here at [hospital name], "Save the Tatas."

On Tuesday 9/22/15, I phoned [Human Resources] and inquired if the breast cancer t-shirt slogan was approved by the hospital administration. Use of that phrase is concerning, perhaps questionable for several reasons. She asked if I had spoken with [manager] from Radiology and suggested maybe she would like to hear another point of view on the slogan. On Wednesday the t-shirt signs were still posted at the hospital building time clocks, but I hadn't spoken again with [Human Resources].

On Friday 9/25/15, I had the chance to stop by [radiology manager's] office for a brief visit in the morning. She did say the slogan was approved, not only by administration but by marketing as well. Radiology had polled the slogan thru some of their patients and she stated it had been well received. I did tell her I found the slogan troubling. For instance, a few years back a t-shirt was made to honor me in a walk by friends- it was not a work-related function. It was difficult to express my true feelings about it to a friend who thought it was great and really excited about doing something for me. In light of that, patients might not reveal an unfavorable opinion on a slogan to someone delivering their care. I explained to [her], such phrases for myself and others like me are similar to pulling a Band-Aid off, reopening a wound every time they are tossed around. When was the last time another cancer was so callously discussed? It is simply not done. She said she sympathized, but the phrase was properly approved. At that point, I had to leave because I was about to cry.

Imagine 1 in 8 women walking through our doors, seeing the slogan and having that same reaction. That would be a 12.5% (or more- considering their families) business lost if they decided to go elsewhere. Cancer is not amusing or cute. It is serious. It can be deadly. When an organization twists a serious topic to make it more fun, comfortable or marketable- that should make us pause.

That afternoon I stopped by your office where you confirmed, indeed the slogan was approved by administration and marketing. The slogan may be approved, but I would hope this letter might enlighten others how it could be inappropriate, especially to be worn in a professional atmosphere. Using words like the slogan (or other euphemisms for breasts) would be poorly received if directed at a patient during clinical exam by a physician or nurse, yet we have them screen-printed on a shirt with the facility logo?

People might innocently misuse phrases or misunderstand something, until they are educated further. Unfortunately education also comes from debilitating personal life experiences that can change our point of view forever. Perhaps I am sensitive on the topic, but we should all be sensitive- especially to our patients diagnosis and disease processes.

In the past I held my opinion about the t-shirts and just didn't buy one. There were emails regarding the [breast cancer] event sponsored by [corporate] a while back. Sure it was a fund raiser to benefit breast cancer, but again- would a physician or nurse say that to a patient? Then why as an organization is it permitted? Just because other people in our society do it in their personal lives and groups does not make it acceptable in a professional atmosphere.

Please consider how many people may not be comfortable with these cute, catchy commercialized phrases used in our culture. There was a standard one family had for their children: would you wear it to church, grandparent's home or school? If not, then don't wear it. Does the slogan reflect a professional image and accurately represent the facility to our patients and community? How many of our male coworkers will purchase and wear the t-shirts while on shift? Are the males uncomfortable wearing said approved t-shirt? How are the shirts perceived by patients? Is the slogan acceptable given our recent compliance training?

I understand decisions are made every day and being one person, just a nurse, I can do nothing about them. Staying silent in the past has only led to this moment of disappointment in the chosen and approved slogan at my own place of work. My hope is that by sharing these thoughts, others may understand and appreciate another point of view going forward.

Undoubtedly, you've seen coverage of a celebrity who has breast cancer or is going through preventative operations due to family history. While it's sad so many people have to deal with cancer, doing it publicly must be a challenge. Even though famous people have access to some of the best care, they are also balancing a personal life and career. Having the ability to fly anywhere and see their choice of physicians, they don't divulge the nitty-gritty, dirty details because they need to remain marketable after they complete their treatment. In an effort to get back to the business of entertainment, they put on a happy face and seem to quickly recover. They don't live like the ordinary person who works an hourly job on their feet to bring home food, clothes for the kids, and afford a healthcare plan. The portrayal of their cancer treatment may lead people to think it's easy. Spoiler alert—it's not.

Another irritant is the coverage of research results given in brief news clips. Every so often, especially in late September and into October, headlines proclaim researchers somewhere found links to cancer if you ingest this, live here, or do that. The stories don't tell you all the pertinent details like how big the study was and whether subjects were human or animal, and they don't tell you how much contact the subjects had over time with the carcinogen. There's just enough information to tease, get attention, and raise anxiety for the general population, and usually end with a disclaimer that more study is needed.

Is it any wonder I'm jaded about the whole pinkified mess?

Breast cancer was no gift or blessing, but it did reveal the true relationships in my life. While awareness campaigns were helpful in the past, that ribbon was also abused. The oversaturation and commercialization are an assault on the senses, especially to those who struggle with the lasting effects of breast cancer, the treatment, or those who are terminal. Cancer doesn't discriminate based on the pocket-book or vocation, but money does buy access to the best care. Countless hours of broadcasting are devoted to silly amuse-ment like "reality shows," while years of scientific study are reduced to thirty-second info-blurbs on news broadcasts. What a disservice to researchers and the audience, perhaps because the content was uncomfortable and not as likely to grab ratings.

Over the years, my *give a shit* got busted. Cancer changed me. Maybe if I hadn't had cancer twice, I wouldn't be as passionate. While I have always been rather social and willing to help anyone out, I'm less likely to tolerate slackers, liars, and bullies. Words fly out of my mouth when common courtesy, safety, and principles are ignored. It can be a curse at times. Go ahead, ask anyone who really knows me, and they'll tell you why I'm not invited to some meetings. (Sometimes people just don't want to hear the truth.)

15

MY SHIT DON'T STINK

My first official attempt at sharing my experiences through writing was actually a contest prompt in the fall of 2012 submitted to a magazine ("The Day that Changes My Life."). It took a few weeks to create, and then a few of my friends edited the piece for grammar and content. I sent it off electronically to some high falutin' muckety muck's mailbox. I had been hopeful about my entry, but it was a nationwide women's magazine and I shouldn't have been surprised at the response. Via e-mail, they thanked me for my contest submission; however, another person's work was chosen. It was meant to be that way so that I would complete the bigger work that you hold in your hands right now.

Some of the material that follows may be a slight repeat for you. It is included as submitted for authenticity, the condensed version of my life up to 2012. Should anyone want to publish it now, you'll have to ask nicely. Kidding. Maybe.

In a matter of months, I'd shaved my head, started a tattoo collection, and began doing some serious drugs.

It was a hectic time, just a few weeks before Christmas

2003. My husband was working full time, a daughter in third grade, a son in preschool, and I was four months into practical nursing school. Thinking back, I still ask—what happened? They say it was probably years in the making, but I'll never really know.

Your mind may be racing, jumping to conclusions. This chick went radically off the deep end, didn't she? The truth is not pretty, not as exciting as you might imagine: suddenly I was a card-carrying member to a club no one wants to join. No one in my family had been through this; I was a non-smoker and a healthy, young female, except for the pesky breast with cancer. That was the end of Me 1.0 as the world knew her.

To make informed decisions, I started surfing the internet for answers. My husband thought I was obsessed with the cancer. Maybe, but if I knew the worst-case scenario, anything else was better, right?

Knowing I'd lose my hair, I had my curly mid-back length hair cut shorter and shorter until it started to fall out. About two weeks after chemotherapy started, we went to the barber who shaved my head, then refused payment, saying, "No charge." I don't like to cry because then I can't breathe and, really, breathing is good. But I broke down and cried—not because of the hair loss, but how unfair it all was.

There was no wig that could compare to my natural hair. Seriously, a web search for a wig of Medusa hair yields pages of Halloween costumes. That hair could be unruly, big, and bushy at times, but it was mine. With nursing school, I chose to wear do-rags, being more afraid of a wig falling off and freaking out a patient, than being honest with people about my "follicularly challenged" state. I did vow, and I've kept my word to this day, to never complain about my hair again. After all that, I appreciate a Bad Hair Day, because a No Hair Day can be very chilly and complicated.

The hair loss was only one of the many possible side effects of chemotherapy (chemo). Just saying chemo makes people shudder, visions of gaunt faces and bald heads. Patients get sick because chemo attacks fast replicating cells —like cancer—but also the hair, stomach, and intestines, which explains the vomiting, diarrhea, and mouth sores too. Whoops, too much information? Sorry, but it's the truth and cancer isn't pretty and pink all the time.

If you don't like needles, I highly recommend a medi-port —easier on the patient and clinic staff to just plug in when veins are hard to find.

I should mention chemo-pause. Hot flashes, sweating, and the menstrual cycle stopped for a while due to chemo. Really, the no cycle thing was nice, but I could've done without the power surges.

With radiation therapy, I got some free tats. At radiation simulation, they marked me for the 33 intense tanning sessions with pinpoint tattoos. For almost 2 months, there was Sharpie marker with clear waterproof dressings on my chest up to my neck. To hide the marks, I wore mock-neck, short-sleeve tops during summer in Oklahoma. Hot much? YES! The drive to treatment was actually longer than it took for the treatments to be administered. I completed radiation with only a couple complications: redness and tender skin.

Everything had gone well. By fall of 2004, I was done with treatment, had the port removed, and was back to work. My hair, which resembled duck fuzz at the start of radiation, had grown to a short, curly, peppered chic look.

Cancer statistics give a 5-year survival rate, so I made a 5-year plan to complete a Bachelor of Science in Nursing. In May 2008, I graduated with my BSN. In December 2008, I celebrated 5 years of "no evidence of disease." My husband and the kids ordered 5 bouquets delivered to me at work. It was a milestone in my personal cancer history in regard to applications for insurance and benefits.

Over the next few years, there were a few concerns about a lump or redness; fortunately, they weren't cancer. In the fall of 2010, my oncologist and I agreed the mammograms every 6 months over 7 years showed I was stable. For Me 2.0, it was time to transition to yearly follow-up visits.

Unfortunately, I found another lump only 4 months later. It was invasive ductal carcinoma again, but slightly different from the first breast cancer. Not a recurrence, a new primary tumor.

Statistically, 1 in 8 women will have breast cancer in her lifetime. I should have been playing the lottery instead. Being diagnosed a second time changed my life plans again, and the update to Me 3.0 began.

We planned for a mastectomy of the cancer side, prophylactic mastectomy of the other breast, and delayed breast reconstruction. For years, I'd had horrible period cramps and debated a hysterectomy. An ultrasound showed my right ovary was enlarged. Trouble? No cancer there, but they did find endometriosis during surgery, and the hysterectomy reduced the chance of recurrence since the tumor was slightly estrogen receptor positive. Chemotherapy would start after healing from the surgeries.

There is nothing like being on the cusp of turning 40, a big year to be celebrated in a big way. I'd planned to travel with my high school friends for our annual get together, but found out I'd be otherwise occupied with treatment. Even though I was off work from March to October, my only "trip" was to the hospital when my white count dipped too low, Neutropenia. Food was good, but no fresh fruit or veggies allowed, also had to wear protective gloves and a mask when venturing out of my room. With no concierge to schedule a concert or outing, I amused myself by writing parody lyrics about the experience for friends online.

People said, "I know how you feel," but I'm not sure they do really. Having a scare with a questionable mammogram is not the same experience of an actual cancer diagnosis. Remember how self-conscious you were about your appearance as a teen? Puberty was hard, sure, but having your breasts amputated and being bald really sucked! The physical and emotional pain of mastectomy and reconstruction can't be compared to elective breast enhancement. They are vastly different experiences, like comparing apples and oranges or grapefruit and melons—pick your favorite fruit euphemism for breasts.

Without hair and a chest, the morning routine gets somewhat quicker. No washing, conditioning, blow drying, or styling hair. Legs and arm pits don't have to be shaved. No bra. I literally shaved off 20 minutes! Think about it, you usually don't worry about your hair matching your outfit. Without hair, you have to consider which do-rag, scarf or hat to pair with an outfit. The wardrobe gets complicated too. If you got it, flaunt it; if you don't, camouflage it. Layered clothes, scarves, and vests helped me feel like people wouldn't be attracted to stare at what was missing.

No chemo-pause in 2011; it was real menopause after the hysterectomy. I should have worked in Vegas! Flinging layers of clothes on and off so fast, your head would spin!

Speaking of Vegas, people wonder about breast reconstruction: Are you gonna get big ones? At least you get some free perky boobs out of it! Big? Mmm, hardly—you don't really get to choose how big you can go, your body chooses because the chest muscles only stretch so far. And free? Ha! There was a price paid, but how can you quantify all a person goes through to get some free boobs after cancer?

There are several options for breast reconstruction after

mastectomy. I chose tissue expanders with exchange to sili-
cone implant prosthesis. I may look normal on the outside,
but these new girls (Breasts 4.0) are nothing like the originals
(Breasts 1.0 or even Breasts 2.0 after lumpectomy). After
mastectomy (that was my Breast-less 3.0 stage), there is loss
of tissue, sensation, and the nipples. Oh, the nipple
complexes can be tattooed or reconstructed, but they are
aesthetic only. I actually fear having my breasts exposed or
injured because I might not feel it happen. Just think of the
Mrs. Doubtfire cooking scene. Scary huh?

People think they know what breast cancer is, but they
really have no idea how ugly pink can be. Breast cancer is not
the good or easy cancer. There are no good cancers. They all
suck. There are different types of breast cancer, and rarely do
people share the same tumor characteristics. A person with
breast cancer at the age of 72 is not the same as a 32 year old.
Treatments vary with the individual, the stage, and the
cancer's origin among other things. A person with a diagnosis
of "in situ" or pre-cancer may be advised to have lumpectomy
or mastectomy. Of course, there are those lucky patients who
get the cancer trifecta: surgery (lumpectomy or mastectomy),
chemo, and radiation.

I'll admit to some anger issues associated with the day
that changed my life. Why did I get cancer? Why did I get it
again? Why do people choose to abuse their bodies and not
get cancer or other diseases? Why do some people turn away
after they find out you have cancer, while others hold you up
and continue to when you need it most? In the midst of the
chaos, it hurts to think how much cancer takes from you.
Addressing my own issues will remain a work in progress my
whole life.

One question people ask that instantly fires me up is: Did
they get it all?

What does that mean? Think about what I've shared and

how you would feel with that question. Did they get it all? Please don't ask that, EVER! To have cancer, go through treatment, and still possibly have it inside—like a ticking bomb—just adds fuel to the fear constantly burning in the back of the mind.

Every fall, stores are full of pink-ribboned items—a portion of the proceeds might go to this, that, or another organization. After experiencing breast cancer, those pink ribbons become a sad reminder. Been there, done that, and been given way too many t-shirts.

Since that day in December of 2003, there are times when life seems normal and I can forget about what we've been through for a few hours. I'll never be Me 1.0 again. I hope those glitches, the 2.0 and 3.0 have been solved, because life with Me 4.0 is going well, but I'll always feel stalked.

I've heard: You're so brave. You're so strong.

Let's agree to disagree. I just don't see myself that way. There are times you do what you have to, to live. What are the alternatives if you don't do everything possible? Would you just throw up your arms and give up? No, you wouldn't. You'd give it all you've got and then some especially when people depend on you. I'm a wife, mom, daughter, sister, aunt, friend, nurse, and more.

Strange as it sounds, I voluntarily got cut up, poisoned, and burned to live. If you saw Me 3.0 out that year, it must have been a really good day. Only my family and closest friends saw the real deal. Would I do it again if I had to? Yes, because I want to be a little old lady wearing a red hat that knits, bakes cookies for her grandkids, and talks to her cat. YES! Actually, no to the cat, I'm allergic, so throw in a Chihuahua as a substitute please. And let's change the red hat to hot pink, and make it sparkly.

16

YOU GOTTA BE SHITTIN' ME

This is the soundtrack chapter to my story. Initially, I'd written some music-related material about my cancer experience. It was rather dark, so I shelved the project. The music-related idea resurfaced after the kids and I watched a movie on TV. It had a great musical score, complete with singing and dancing, and told a cool story (and I'd liked the lead actor for years).

I'm going to encourage you to take a brief potty break. Empty your bladder, because I do not want the blame if you should have an accident after revealing the inspirational movie title. Go ahead, but if you insist you are good, then read on, but you have been warned.

This is no joke. If you laugh, that's fine, I understand. From my journal dated 3-17-15: I have decided to go back to writing my book idea and incorporating music. Got the idea from *Rock of Ages*. Tom Cruise was mmm-memorable...

Julianne Hough, Catherine Zeta Jones, Tom Cruise, and several other stars were featured, and it convinced me that my musical story idea made sense.

What follows is just a fraction of the music that really

relates to my life and would make a great mix tape or one kick-ass live show. Picture it in lights: *CA CA, the musical* or just two giant sparkly pink poop emoji.

"Honey, I've just won tickets to *CA CA*!"

"Date night: we're seeing some shitty musical—seriously, it's called *CA CA*!"

If there were one song that could describe your attitude, your outlook, what would it be? Maybe the entire song doesn't fit, but a verse or the chorus does? It perfectly captures how you feel, what you're going through, where you've been.

Music is magical. Some songs are so eloquent in their phrasing, and when coupled with the right instrumentation, there's an emotional response. Certain pieces of music can remind us of people, places, and times that are stored in the deepest recesses of our minds. Just a few notes can release memories that rush to the surface of our consciousness. Think back and you can recall a song from way back when, like from your prom or that hymn at your grandma's funeral.

When I hear songs, I really like to listen to the lyrics. Try to listen to a new song or an older song that you may not know all the lyrics to. You might be surprised by what people are singing sometimes! Some of what follows might fall in that category.

For brevity (and copyright reasons), I'm not going to directly quote songs or write out lyrics. You can easily check out various internet sites for that, *or* you can go directly to the songs themselves. I highly encourage you to give them a listen and try to identify the specific verses that fit in my *CA CA*.

In our early years of marriage, we were just starting out, a young couple stationed away from family with the challenges of military life, college, one vehicle, and taking on new adult responsibilities at age twenty. By today's standards, we were poor, but happy with our life together. Our love would conquer all (and it has). That innocence of the early years was like Sonny & Cher in "I Got You Babe."

So there we were, a few years later with work, school, and the kids' activities that kept us busy. But we were living the dream with our little Tink and Bubba. "She's Come Undun" by The Guess Who fits after the cancer bomb was dropped on me at the doctor's office. All those people who denied the possibility of cancer, saying "Nah, can't be, too young…" didn't prepare me for what I heard.

Then there were many appointments, procedures, and treatments. Doctors, nurses, and many other healthcare professionals would direct, interact, and play specific parts in the drama. Fade in "See me. Feel me. Touch me. Heal Me…" by The Who.

At times, I was pretty overwhelmed. There is no GPS (global positioning system) type of guide for cancer, or life for that matter. I was unsure about what to do at times since I didn't know anyone with personal experience similar to mine. I was a grown-ass independent woman and yet so much was suddenly beyond my control. If you want to talk in terms of life's journey, having cancer was an obstacle, a roadblock, the ultimate dropped call, or shitty cell service. So you have to re-route. It was strange how often I would hear just what I needed. One song was about being blue, but sticking it out and weathering the storm. Jo Dee Messina's "Bring on the Rain" inspired me. I'd belt it out while driving alone in the minivan and I'd feel better. (Recalculating…Drive…)

People talk about how life is too short. Yes, you have to work, live, eat, and raise your family. It's sad to think about, but many of us are easily replaced on the job. We need to do more living, enjoying those people who make you laugh, and taking time to do things on that bucket list. Find a little joy every single day. You never know whether you'll get another opportunity, so it's no surprise that I'd hear Tim McGraw's ballad, "Live Like You Were Dying" and feel like he was singing to me.

Breast cancer was an attack that came out of nowhere, no family history for someone so young and healthy. During radiation, I imagined any remaining microscopic cancer cells being knocked out. It was the last part of the active treatment plan. As I waited on the table, I was focused on getting it all done and beating the cancer beast. So, Mister Radiation Technician, like Pat Benatar sang, "Hit Me with Your Best Shot."

There were so many people who cared, prayed, and sent cards and packages over the months of diagnosis and treatment. They stepped up and made me feel like I was living Martina McBride's song, "Blessed."

Then when you're all done with active treatment, you graduate. Now what? The doctors check every so often for *no evidence of disease*. You're a different person after cancer and may not have the abilities or desire to resume your "old" ways. Often you feel sad, mad, bad, or glad, possibly all at the same time on the same day? The increased anxiety with any strange aches or pains, symptoms, the various tests, and the follow-up appointments *is* the new normal. You discover you can easily relate to 4 Non Blondes in "What's Up?"

When I hit my five-year diagnosis date, a number of people were in on a big secret to mark the occasion. My husband planned delivery of numerous flower bouquets and my coworkers threw a party. It was a "Celebration" like Kool and the Gang sang, and we were happy to mark a big milestone.

Life was good. There were a few scares, but they turned out okay. When I found the second lump, my heart sank. It felt like I had a stalker. A dark encounter was back from the past to turn my life inside out despite all of my efforts to live well. How is that fair? We would do everything to resist it *again*. I wasn't about to give up and sounded my protest with "Jar of Hearts" by Christina Perri.

The first cancer experience had left me with a few physical scars and some emotional baggage. When I knew all that would have to happen again, the surgeries and chemo, I had some dark days about the many things I couldn't control. Cancer isn't pretty or packaged in a shiny ribbon. It robs. It takes away the breasts, the uterus, the hair, the stomach contents, and life as you know it. It hurts. And the second time, you have more scars, more pain, more isolation. It disfigures, and makes you physically and psychologically vulnerable. It changes people, makes one feel outcast. To me, Skillet's "Monster" accurately depicts living with cancer.

So often we get caught up in the everyday stuff and stay busy, lose touch, or just don't have time to meet up. When something bad happens, you see people pitch in to help out. Some people you'd expect to be there just won't, because they can't hack it.

Who's there? Your partner, your kids, your faith. "I'll Stand By You" by the Pretenders fits to describe a relationship with a mate or your children, because it's about backing someone up no matter what the odds or issue. It also fits my relationship with God. He gets me, understands me, and is somehow always there for me. I probably don't say it enough but I'm so glad *He's got my back*. *Always*. Only by His grace am I still here today.

Cancer unites, but it also divides. People are scared for you. It hits too close to home for them. They try to be supportive, but their good intention comes off badly in their words or actions. No Doubt sang it best—it might be better if they "Don't Speak."

The surgery, the chemo, and the side effects can be debilitating. If only you could get away or do something productive. There was so much I couldn't do. It was frustrating. Normal household chores, working, even eating certain things were off limits. I learned to knit. I read books. I watched movies. I tried to cope. I enjoyed the Ramones, "I Wanna Be Sedated." I even wrote parody lyrics when hospitalized because I had a little too much time to think about my current situation.

There are people who truly understand what you're going through. They are the ones who have been there, done that, and got the t-shirt. Caregivers can see what you've been though, but they haven't been to that dark place themselves. The Mighty Mighty Bosstones happy-go-lucky sounding tune "The Impression That I Get" was used as the intro music to a popular home video show, where people frequently got hit in the private parts, fell over, or knocked down a hill. The intro used music only, whereas the song lyrics reflect the *oh that had to hurt, thank God that wasn't me, and don't know what I'd do* feeling when pondering someone else's misfortune. The song lyric's irony as a theme for the show is not lost on me.

You can't compare an augmentation of the breast to mastectomy with reconstruction. They are two entirely different things. Don't compare your "scare" to my reality either. Your "scare" is valid, but will never be the same as amputation of breasts, loss of hair, loss of ovaries, and years of medication to prevent cancer coming back. These are two different experiences. The reality is all of us will meet our demise, some sooner than others, and it sucks when people seem to minimize what you're having to deal with on a daily basis. Trite affirmations given on any life situation, when that person doesn't know jack squat about the treatment or prognosis, just piss me off, so until you've walked the walk, zip it. I was able to see the Foo Fighters perform "These Days." LOVED IT! Best concert ever.

I had a posse of friends from years back. They were

dubbed the pinklings. They phoned, texted (the tinklings of the pinklings), mailed cards, and sent a fabulous concert disc of the one and only P!nk (her performance amazed me, is there anything she can't do?). "Raise Your Glass" never fails to bolster my confidence or cheer me up, and that's why it's the ring tone for when my girls call. Cheers ladies!

Just when I needed a bit of encouragement, I found strength and confidence when the theme from *Rocky* ("Gonna Fly Now") played on the radio as I was on the road the day of my reconstruction surgery (and I happened to be wearing grey sweat pants and a hoodie). That picture on the cover— that's me on that very day, and I'm still laughing about it too.

Several doctors coordinated my care after cancer (PCP, oncologist, plastic surgeon) and I had a rough year as reconstruction started. There was a reaction to the flu shot at the injection site, hospitalization for pneumonia and cardiomyopathy workup, and several antibiotic prescriptions for possible infection related to the implants. I would journal thoughts, feelings, and trials. It was helpful to process and then aided in recalling my experiences when my writing project picked up again. The passages revealed the emotional drain, some clinical notations, lots of humorous anecdotes, even a bit of venom. For me, the song "Breathe" by Anna Nalick summed up the creative process. You can experience something, record it, reflect on it later, and realize it is what it is—it's in the past. It can redefine you, and whether it's positive or negative is determined by you.

Things didn't work out with reconstruction. I'm happy for the people who have done well, but in the end, it wasn't for me. Some people may not understand and think it was a move backward or a failure. People tend to be uncomfortable and question what they haven't experienced. After years of trying to regain some semblance of my real breasts, the process had run its disappointing course, with the lack of

sensation and coolness to the touch, among other complications. The decision to be my imperfect authentic self without
the breast implants and pain was a relief. It was a realization
that I didn't have to live up to any expectations or need
approval from anyone to be myself. Imagine Dragons' "On
Top of the World" resonates with the physical and emotional
healing I'd finally achieved.

In January 2017, I saw a post on Facebook questioning
what would you do if you knew you would not fail. Easy—
complete my writing. Get it out there. Help someone.
Someone has to tell it like it is. Why not me? In "Galileo,"
the Indigo Girls' harmony and message relate how life may
never be perfect despite our effort, but we can use the experience and share the story in order to grow.

The development of *CA CA* was an investment, a great
deal of thought and time examining myself. In spite of everything I endured, I think I've blossomed. Think of the simple
yet complex dandelion. Some see the seed as a beginning or a
wish, the green leaves as troublesome weeds, the flower given
as a token of love. What about their tenacity? Tiny bits of
fuzz plucked from a stem are carried by the wind to places
unknown. With ample nutrients, they root and flourish to
begin anew. Seek out Alanis Morissette's hit "Hand In My
Pocket" to consider your own nature.

Well, my friend, you've got my *CA CA* on your hands
right now. We got down to business with facts (statistics, clinical explanations), added in the party (humor, most of it at my
own expense), and the casual (brutal honesty from the depths
of my heart). When asked to describe me, those closest to me
replied: genuine, forthright, tenacious, incredibly loyal, a
maverick, a dark horse that comes off as unassuming with an
unapologetic commitment to corny humor. Here's the *CA CA*
equation: zero family history, pink cancer to the second
power plus chemo plus radiation minus body parts, multiple

reconstructions divided by a factor of time with a variable amount of sparkling wit. Proof positive—I am a human mullet.

As this book nears completion, we come to the present time. It should wrap up with a nearly happily-ever-after type song. That's where I'm at right now, a good place to be. But not a track that's over the top, with blue skies all the time and sugary sweet. I need a song that acknowledges life's many challenges, reflecting and appreciating the value in all the events—both the bad and the good. I'll leave you with OneRepublic, "I Lived."

17

I AM SO DONE WITH THIS SHIT

For the years I'd avoided writing about my experience, I'd also avoided my own conflict resolution. Back in high school English class, we studied literary conflict. There was man versus man, nature, society, technology, or himself. The character was ultimately forced to address an issue, and then deal with it by some sort of change, insanity, or death.

Writing was a therapeutic process. After reviewing my journals, blogs, notes, and previous drafts over many cups of coffee, I'd found some peace. With time, I'd changed, mostly for the better. There had been enough conflict: woman versus nature (cancer), technology (treatment), society (pink exploitation, discomfort over cancer), man (shitheads, bean counters), and self (fear of cancer, overcoming anxiety and image issues). If my experience has done anything to help someone else in their treatment, I'm glad to have finally shared it. After all, I'm the irrepressible Authentic M who gets shit done.

There are so many people I want to acknowledge, but I

refrained from using names in the book to maintain the privacy of others. I could tell so many more stories that involve family, in-laws, and friends over the years, but I shan't at this juncture. So how do you recognize those amazing people without naming names? Nicknames. That's how.

MM -N- RH 4ever. Always.

Tink and Bubba- you schmoopaloos are the bestest kids ever. Bevvy loves you.

Thanks to my parents and siblings for the love, in presents and presence. The people that would and have bent over backwards, picked me up and gave me the pajamas off their back.

Gratitude to my in-laws and extended family for their kindness and support.

Here's to one more day above the roses, cheers to my girls, the EEW pinklings.

My local posse: Yin to my Yang, neighbor from the hood, Nighthawk's buddy, dance parents, band parents, teachers, people at the coffee shop that kept me caffeinated (or decaffeinated as need be), coworkers, my doctors, their staff...

If you happen to be one of those whom I unfortunately forget to mention either by nickname or by "groupie" status —I'm grateful for the years of friendship, care, and prayers.

Thanks to Ms. J (and her FOM discount) my five-year goal is finally completed (okay, so I'm a bit late!).

Here is my long-distance dedication (imagine Casey Kasem's radio voice or mine as I try to imitate him).

The Irrepressible Authentic M writes: *Years ago my life changed in a single afternoon. I did what I had to, even though I didn't want to at times. The experience changed me, made me a different person who'd gained perspective and finally some peace. If I could help just one person with their own frustration and heartache by sharing my story, I'm glad to have done it. I had help along the way from many people—some I knew personally, some I didn't adequately express my gratitude to, and some who said my experience helped them realize it was time to take control of their health. I'd like to say thank you, I'm sorry, and you're welcome. In appreciation and encouragement to them, please share "Unwritten" by Natasha Bedingfield.*

A LOAD OF SHIT: REFERENCES/SOURCES

Cancer Stat Facts: Female Breast Cancer Percent of New Cases by Age Group. *National Cancer Institute at the National Institutes of Health.* Retrieved November 25, 2017 from https://seer.cancer.gov/statfacts/html/breast.html

Christensen, Barbara Lauritsen and Elaine Oden Kockrow. *Foundations of Nursing.* St Louis: Mosby, 2003. Print. (p. 167)

Diethylstilbestrol (DES) and Cancer. (Reviewed October 5, 2011). *National Cancer Institute at the National Institutes of Health.* Retrieved July 25, 2017 from https://www.cancer.gov/abot-cancer/causes-prevention/risk/hormones/des-fact-sheet

Love, Susan M. M.D., and Karen Lindsey. *Dr. Susan Love's Breast Book. 5th ed.,* Philadelphia: 1st Da Capo Press Perseus ed., 2010. Ibook edition.

McCance, Kathryn L. and Sue E. Huether. *Pathophysiology The Biologic Basis for Disease in Adults and Children.* St Louis: Elsevier Mosby, 2006. Print. (p.848 figure 23-55)

Nettina, Sandra M. *Lippincott Manual of Nursing Practice.*

Philadelphia: Lippincott Williams & Wilkins, 2001. Print. (p.802, figure 23-1)

U.S. Breast Cancer Statistics. (Page last modified April 19, 2011). *breastcancer.org.* Retrieved April 19, 2011. http://www.breastcancer.org/symptoms/understand_bc/statistics.jsp

Music

Bedingfield, Natasha. "Unwritten." *Unwritten Single*. Phonogenic/Epic. 2004. NOW21

Benatar, Pat. "Hit Me With Your Best Shot." *Heartbreaker Sixteen Classic Performances.* EMI Records. 1996. Compact Disc. (originally ATV Music Corp. 1980.)

Foo Fighters. "These Days." *Wasting Light*. RCA. 2011. Compact Disc.

The Guess Who. "Undun." *The Guess Who: Greatest Hits*. BMG. 1999. Itunes. (Originally *Canned Wheat*. 1969.)

Imagine Dragons. "On Top of the World." *Night Visions*. KIDinaKORNER/Interscope Records. 2012. Itunes.

Indigo Girls. "Galileo." *Retrospective*. Sony Music. 2000. Compact Disc. (originally on *Rites of Passage*. Jill Music Ltd. 1992)

Kool & the Gang. "Celebration." *Celebration: The Best of Kool & the Gang 1979-1987*. Poly Gram Records. 1994. Compact Disc.

McBride, Martina. "Blessed." *Greatest Hits*. RCA Records. 2001. Compact Disc.

McGraw, Tim. "Live Like You Were Dying." *Greatest Hits Vol 2 Reflected*. 2006. Curb Records, Inc. (originally Warner Tamerlane Publishing Corp. 2004.)

Messina, JoDee. "Bring On The Rain." *Greatest Hits*. Curb Records. 2003. Compact Disc. (originally Mike Curb Records. 2000.)

Mighty Mighty Bosstones. "The Impression That I Get."

The Millenium Collection: The best of the Mighty Mighty Bosstones. The Island Def Jam Music Group. 2005. Itunes.

Morissette, Alanis. "Hand In My Pocket." *Jagged Little Pill (Collector's Edition)*. Maverick Recording Company. 2015. Itunes.

Nalick, Anna. "Breathe(2am)-Single." *Breathe(2AM)-Single*. Sony BMG. 2004. Itunes.

No Doubt. "Don't Speak." *Tragic Kingdom*. Interscope Records. 1995. Compact Disc.

OneRepublic. "I Lived." *Native*. Mosley Music/Interscope Records. 2014. Itunes.

Perri, Christina. "Jar of Hearts." *Love Strong*. Atlantic. 2010. Itunes.

P!NK. "Raise Your Glass." *Raise Your Glass- Single*. LaFace Records. 2010. Itunes.

The Pretenders. "I'll Stand By You." *Last of the Independents*. Sire. 1994. Compact Disc *VH1 Classic The Cuts*.

The Ramones. "I Wanna Be Sedated." *Hey Ho Let's Go-Greatest Hits(Remastered)*. Warner Bros. 2006. Itunes.

Skillet. "Monster." *Awake*. Lava/Ardent/Atlantic. 2009. Itunes.

Sonny & Cher. "I Got You Babe." *Look At Us*. Atco. 1965. Itunes.

The Who. "See Me, Feel Me." *Then and Now (1964-2004)*. Record label. 2004.

4 Non Blondes. "What's up?" *Bigger Better Faster More!* 1993. Interscope. Itunes.

Additional recommended reading or viewing:

Albom, Mitch. *The Five People You Meet In Heaven*. 2003. Hyperion.

breastcancer.org

The Bucket List. Dir. Rob Reiner. 2001. Warner Bros. Warner Home Video.

cancer.org for the American Cancer Society

The Doctor. Dir. Randa Haines. 1991. Warner Bros. Warner Home Video.

The Fault in Our Stars. Dir. Josh Boone. 2014. Twentieth Century Fox Home Entertainment LLC.

Mukherjee, Siddhartha. *The Emperor of All Maladies A Biography of Cancer.* Scribner, 2011.

Olson, James S. *Bathsheba's Breast- Women, Cancer & History*. The Johns Hopkins University Press, 2002.

Pink Ribbons Inc. Dir Lea Pool. 2011. First Run Features.

Rock of Ages. Dir. Adam Shankman. 2012. New Line Cinema. Warner Home Video.

Skloot, Rebecca. *The Immortal Life of Henrietta Lacks*. Gale Group, 2011.

Made in the USA
Middletown, DE
14 March 2023

26726138R00076